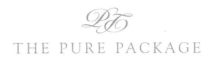

THE PURE PACKAGE

The Balance Diet

Quick & easy recipes to feel healthy & slim

Jennifer Irvine

WEIDENFELD & NICOLSON

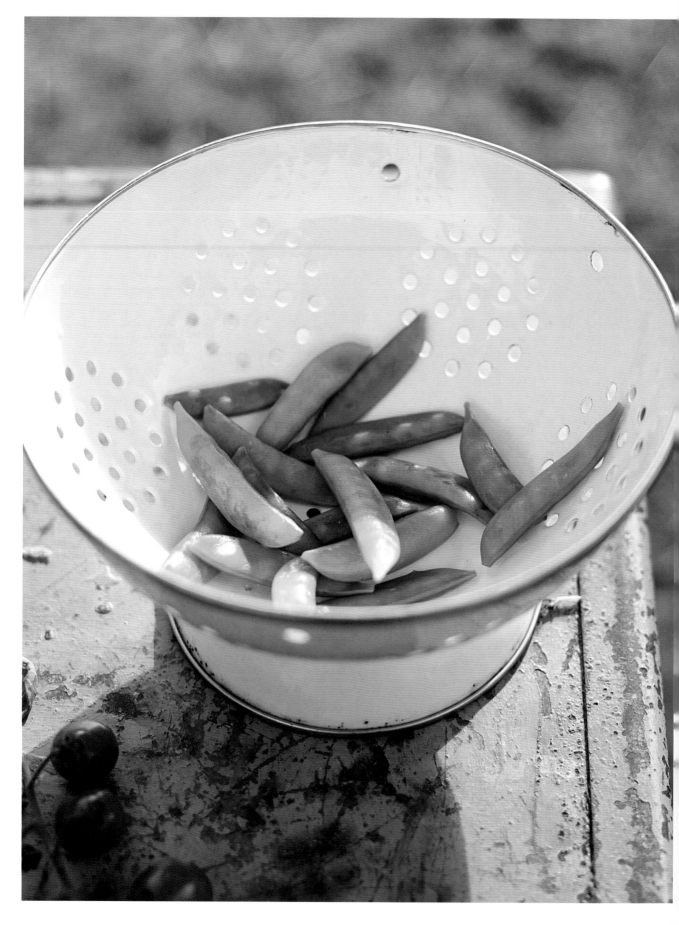

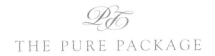

THE PURE PACKAGE

The Balance Diet

First published in Great Britain in 2013
by Weidenfeld & Nicolson, an imprint of
Orion Publishing Group Ltd
Orion House, 5 Upper St Martin's Lane,
London WC2H 9EA
An Hachette UK company

10 9 8 7 6 5 4 3 2 1

A CIP catalogue record for this book is
available from the British Library.

ISBN: 978-0-297-86659-6

Photography by Dan Jones
Design and art direction by Julyan Bayes
Food styling by Lucy O'Reilly
Prop styling by Tamzin Ferdinando
Project edited by Kate Wanwimolruk
Copy-edited by Emily Sweet
Proofread by Jennifer Wheatley
Index by Hilary Bird

Printed and bound in China

The Orion Publishing Group's policy is to use papers that
are natural, renewable and recyclable products and made
from wood grown in sustainable forests. The logging and
manufacturing processes are expected to conform to the
environmental regulations of the country of origin.

www.orionbooks.co.uk

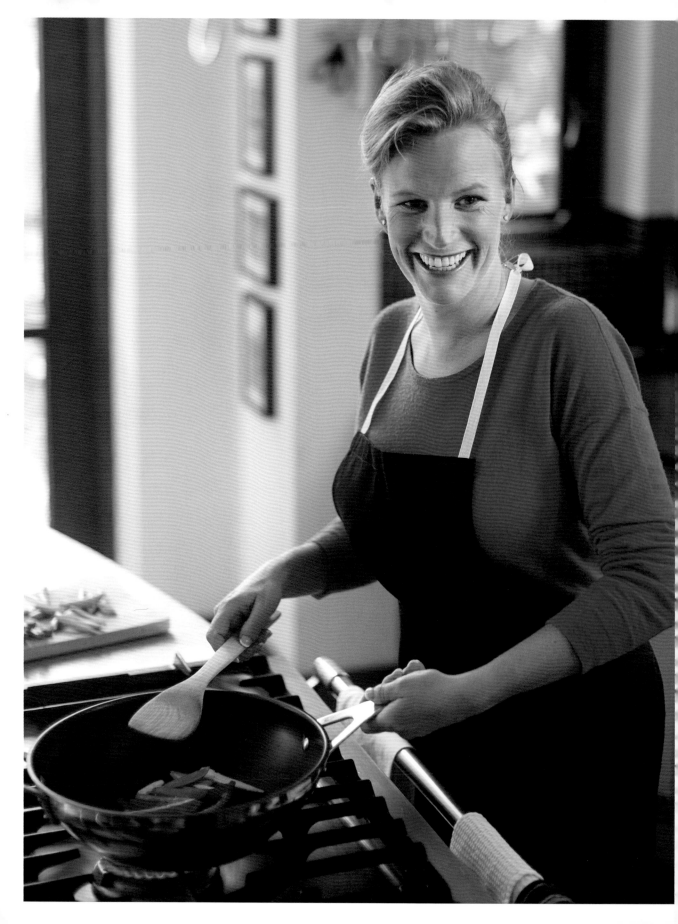

TIME
is the thing I am most short of, so when I cook at home I need quick and easy recipes that don't compromise on flavour and goodness.

I am your typical busy, multi-tasking, working mum – but I don't believe that means I have to let healthy eating slip. And so it was with excitement that I embarked on writing this book, the aim being simple: to share everyday recipes to help make your path to losing weight just that bit easier and more satisfying.

The key to slim waistlines and feeling good is eating the right proportions. Portion control is the backbone of The Pure Package's philosophy. You could be eating all the right things but still be overweight and lethargic just because your ratio of key food groups is slightly off. Here, you will find recipes that are nutritionally balanced, easy to mix and match and, most importantly, fuss-free. I have also included recipe variations (where possible) and practical, time-saving tips to make your meal planning a little more streamlined – as well as setting out an easy-to-follow 14-day healthy eating plan.

With busy lives you need convenience and flexibility. This is why the majority of recipes have been made to serve two – you can easily double or triple quantities. I urge you to make extra portions so that you can delve into my concept of 'upcycling'. Essentially leftovers 'rebooted', upcycling is not about reheating and eating the same meal again; but rather creating new dishes to be enjoyed in their own right.

By following *The Balance Diet* plan and cooking my recipes, you will gain vigour, lose weight and maintain your ideal size. But most of all, I hope you will enjoy the vibrant ingredients, textures and flavours the recipes have to offer.

Jennifer Irvine
Founder, The Pure Package

GOLDEN GUIDELINES

When I was setting up The Pure Package, I was overwhelmed by just how much science is associated with health and nutrition; it seems that we are constantly bombarded by new terminology and research. I wanted to condense all this information into a set of simple rules that encapsulate the core principles for healthy living. These Golden Guidelines will offer a way of eating that gives you control without the need for a calculator.

The rule of palm

At The Pure Package we often have customers who say they eat the right thing, but just too much of it. The key to achieving a healthy body size and strong energy levels is to recognise that *how much* we eat is just as important as *what* we eat.

The Rule of Palm is a straightforward method for determining how much we should be eating for optimal health. Although calorie-counting or weighing your food can be helpful (which is why we have included a calorie breakdown of the recipes in this book on page 216), being too focused on calculations can leave you feeling overwhelmed and seems impractical on a day-to-day basis. Instead, be guided by the size of your palm as a way of working out the portion size that's right for you.

Your meals should consist of three key components: protein, complex carbohydrates, and fruit and vegetables. For a balanced meal, you should fill your plate using the following Rule of Palm formula:

- 1 palm-size portion of protein
- 1 palm-size portion of complex carbohydrates
- 2 palm-size portion of vegetables or fruit

No complex equations, no unfathomable formulas delivered in double-Dutch; just an easy-to-remember, common-sense approach to eating and portion control.

This is science simplified and it really does work. Try it, and I know you'll enjoy the benefits too.

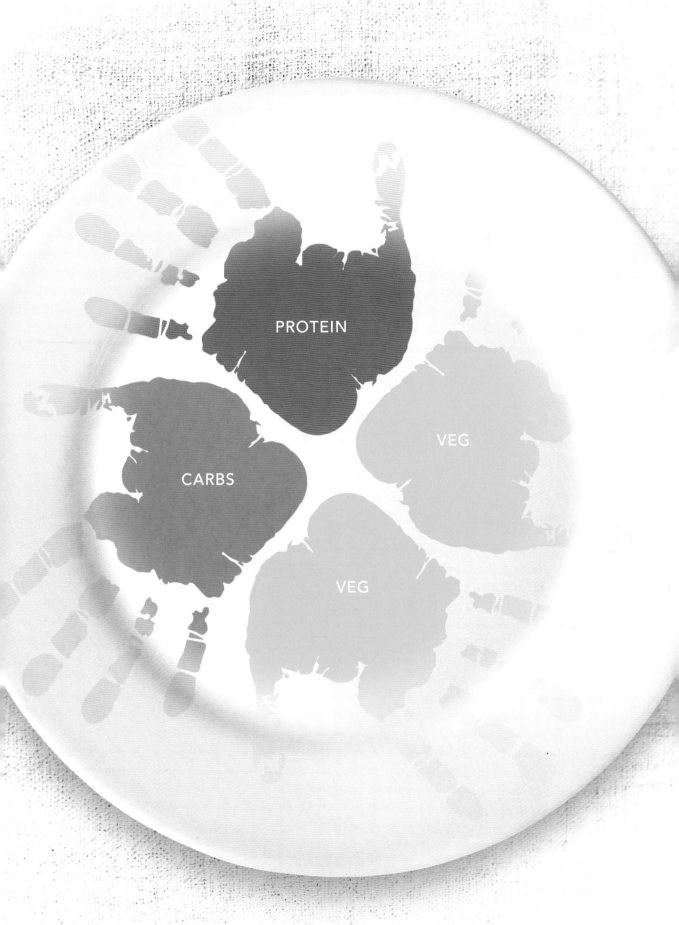

Eat the rainbow

Colour is nature's way of advertising the inherent goodness and nutritional value of food. In their natural state, fruits, vegetables, herbs and spices burst with different coloured hues, reflecting their health-giving properties.

Eating a variety of brightly coloured fruits and vegetables helps to maintain a healthy digestive system, ward off illness and prevent premature ageing. So instead of splashing out on expensive face creams, simply increase your consumption of fruits and vegetables.

Here is a brief breakdown of some of the benefits of eating the rainbow:

- Green – broccoli, cabbage and spinach – contain nutrients including lutein, lycopene, zeaxanthin, folic acid and glucosinolates – all of which have been associated with lowering the risk of cancer

- Orange – carrots, oranges, squashes and sweet potatoes – are high in carotenoids, crucial for maintaining a good immune system and supporting cell repair and healthy vision

- Blue and purple – blueberries, blackberries, grapes and purple sprouting broccoli – are extremely high in antioxidants, promote healthy blood, and are thought to have anti-ageing properties

- Yellow – corn, pineapple and squashes – contain large amounts of bioflavonoids, which fight infection and reduce inflammation

- Red – cherries, strawberries, cranberries and raspberries – contain high levels of anthocyanins, which are thought to be effective in fighting cancer, bacterial infections and neurological diseases

By all means consult a dietitian, nutritionist or other professional, but my advice would be to get sensible, keep it simple, and relish eating colour for its own sake.

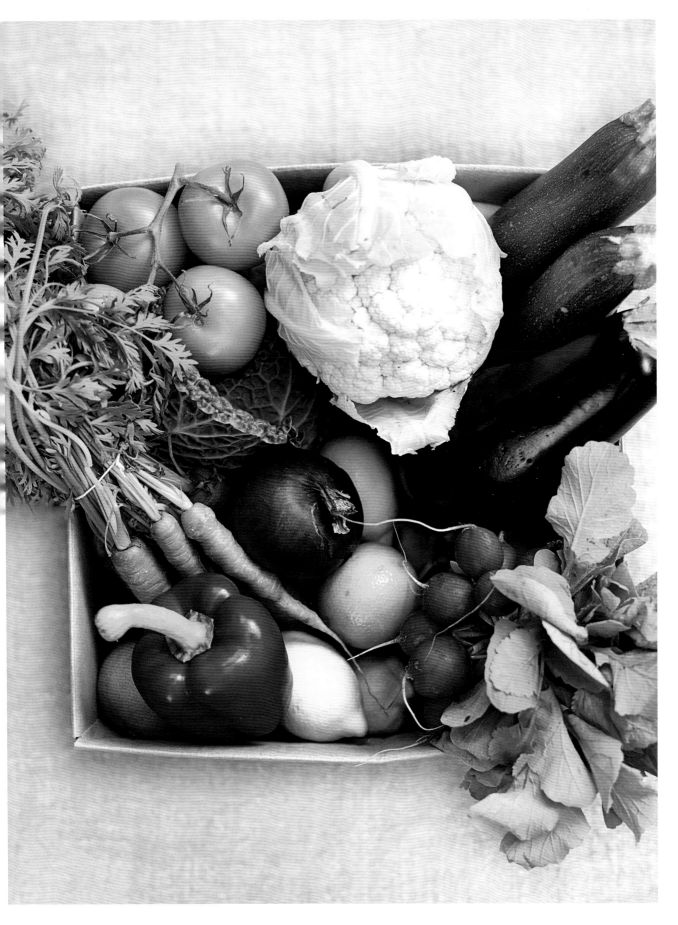

Eat complex carbohydrates

Eating the right carbs plays a vital role in maintaining a healthy diet. Carbohydrates can be defined as organic compounds in plants that are broken down when digested and converted into glucose, which the body uses for energy. However, not all carbohydrates are nutritionally equal and for a healthy diet we need to consume more 'complex carbohydrates', that is, those which release their energy more slowly and keep you feeling full for longer.

Complex carbohydrates are found in whole grains, vegetables and legumes (beans and lentils). However, in this book, when we refer to complex carbs we are talking about whole grains (such as millet, oats, oat bran, wheat germ, barley, wild rice, brown rice, rye, spelt, buckwheat and cornmeal) and skin-on potatoes. The carbohydrates we want to avoid are 'simple carbohydrates', such as white bread, white rice and sugar, which are converted to glucose and released into the bloodstream quickly. This creates peaks and drops in the blood-sugar level, leading to fluctuating energy, cravings and, ultimately, weight gain.

It is safe to assume that the less processing food has undergone, the more complex it is. For example, a grain of wheat: if it has been dehusked, multi-washed, bleached and treated to resemble talcum powder, it is no longer a complex carbohydrate (in spite of the highly complicated journey it has been on). Over-processed foods are stripped not only of nutrients but also of the fibre that our bodies need for effective and efficient digestion.

Complex carbs, when treated well, make really nourishing and satisfying dishes and in this book you will find plenty of recipes that use them to their full potential. The Rule of Palm (see page 8) provides the discipline, enabling us to indulge ourselves in the comfort foods we love, without the guilt. Eating complex carbohydrates is the best way to ensure that your body is getting the fibre and nutrients it needs, as well as indispensable slow-burning energy – delivered as nature intended.

Eat lean protein & essential fats

Protein is crucial for our health and well-being and for a strong body. We need protein, whether it's in the form of a macho-grilled steak over the barbecue, an elegantly steamed piece of fish, or a comforting bowl of chickpea curry.

Consuming lean protein in particular enables our bodies to build, replenish and repair tissue and organs. In this book, when we refer to lean protein, we mean 'complete' proteins, such as poultry, beef, pork, venison and fish. These foods are considered to be complete because they contain all the essential amino acids that need to be included in our daily diet, as our bodies can not produce them. If you prefer not to consume animal protein there are other protein sources you can turn to such as nuts, pulses, mushrooms and tofu that will ensure your diet is well balanced.

Along with protein, we need fats as part of a balanced diet. Fats are a food group we often avoid when trying to banish the pounds. However, not all of them are bad. In fact, because essential fats cannot be produced by our bodies, they are absolutely key to good health if incorporated into our diets sparingly. Each day you should consume a thumb-sized portion of essential fats by eating foods or oils that contain them.

Essential fats fall into two groups, both of which are needed for good health. Omega-6 fatty acids are found in vegetable oils, meat, eggs, avocados, nuts and whole grains. Omega-3 fatty acids are found in oily fish, soy beans, and nuts and seeds (particularly flax seeds and walnuts).

I use groundnut oil, coconut oil and grapeseed oil for cooking because they have a high 'flash' point, meaning they can be heated to a high temperature without losing their beneficial qualities. Olive, hazelnut, sesame, avocado, walnut and pumpkin oil are better enjoyed raw because they have been cold pressed (not exposed to heat during the extraction process), so retain their nutritional value and flavours.

The recipes in this book will encourage you to consume more good fats and oils, and fewer unhealthy ones. The most unhealthy fats are 'trans fats', created when liquid oil is made into a solid fat through a process called hydrogenation. Trans fats can raise your cholesterol and clog arteries, as well as contributing to heart disease and weight gain. Because they are cheap, and give food a longer shelf-life, they are commonly used in processed foods (particularly cakes, pies and ready-made meals). You can avoid trans fats very easily just by eating food as close to its natural state as possible, and by making your own meals and snacks from scratch.

CLEVER SNACKS

It's time to talk about the dietary elephant in the room: snacking. Fundamentally, we need to snack, yet people still seem to ignore this natural urge that is necessary for optimal health.

Across all of our Pure Package food programmes we cannot emphasise enough how important snacking is to achieve consistent energy levels and a healthy body. We all know the value of three well-balanced meals a day, and we need to give the same attention to snacking between mealtimes.

When mid-morning and mid-afternoon come around, we all feel that pang of hunger. This shouldn't be ignored – it is your body's way of telling you that it has hit an energy slump and needs some refuelling. To stop you from reaching for the simplest and easiest solution – more often than not found in the cookie jar – you will need to be organised.

Below are snack suggestions categorised into fruit-based and savoury. Try to have one of each per day, for example, one fruit-based snack mid-morning and one savoury snack mid-afternoon. Pre-prepared snacks are also wonderfully versatile for when you're on the go – simply pack them in an airtight container, and pop into your bag before you go out.

As well as being important sources of nutrients, my snack suggestions will help keep your energy levels steady throughout the day. So now, far from being ashamed of your snacking habit, I urge you to flaunt it!

Fruit-based

Fresh fruit is an ideal mid-morning snack, and if consumed with a handful of nuts or seeds, you will feel full for longer. As well as being packed with protein and essential fats, nuts and seeds slow down the rate at which the fruit's sugars are absorbed by the body, steadying blood-sugar levels. Choose unsalted nuts or seeds and use your palm as a guide for portion size.

There are endless fruit and nut/seed combinations to explore so feel free to experiment. Here are just a few ideas to inspire you:

- Peach and pecans
- Mango and pistachios
- Pineapple and cashew nuts
- Banana and walnuts
- Kiwi fruit and sunflower seeds

Savoury

Like everyone else, my energy levels take another tumble mid-afternoon, so I like to reach for a palm-sized portion of something savoury that won't compromise health and vitality. A protein-rich snack eaten with some carbohydrate or veg for added crunch hits the spot perfectly and keeps energy levels even.

FOR PROTEIN

- Bean-based dips
- Ready-smoked fish
- Cream-cheese dips
- Nut butters
- Avocados
- Cheese

FOR CRUNCH

- Oatcakes
- Toasted rye or spelt bread
- Chopped vegetables (e.g. carrots, celery, cucumber, radishes, sugar snap peas)
- Sliced apple or pear

I urge you to make your own dips, which can be as quick as they are easy. Just choose one of the following protein bases, and mix with one (or more) of the suggested flavour additions. Depending on the consistency you're after, you can either mash them together in a bowl or whizz together until smooth in a blender or food processor. There really is no magic to it, and no formal recipe – just mix, taste, adjust flavours if necessary, and enjoy. Crisp, raw pieces of vegetables are perfect for scooping.

Base protein	Flavour additions
Chickpeas	Freshly squeezed lemon juice
Smoked mackerel	Sun-dried tomato
Half-fat cream cheese or low-fat natural yoghurt	Finely chopped herbs: parsley, basil, coriander, mint
Broad beans	Pesto (see page 96)
Feta cheese	Roasted red pepper
Avocado	Finely chopped chilli
Soya beans	Crushed garlic
Peanut butter	Drizzle of olive oil

UPCYCLING

This imaginative approach to using up leftovers makes preparing lunches and snacks a doddle.

Rather than just recycling the original dish; the idea is to create something new from any leftover component. For example, having enjoyed a smoked mackerel and potato salad today, simply mash some leftover fish with the salad's dressing to produce a moreish pâté for tomorrow's afternoon snack.

The concept of upcycling is also at the crux of the 14-Day Plan on pages 211–213. It enables you to plan your week (or fortnight) so that you have your ingredients cooked and ready to upcycle when you need them. This saves time during the working week when it is hard to find a minute to take a breather, let alone whip up a fully balanced meal.

Throughout the book I have provided upcycling ideas to show you that with just a bit of thought, you can have a whole new dish at the ready in mere minutes. Below are just a few upcycling methods to help you rethink your approach to leftovers.

- Wraps are an easy and practical way to upcycle last night's meal. All you need to do is fill and fold. Opt for wholewheat over white flour wraps and check that they are free of trans fats.

- Open sandwiches allow generous fillings and keep bread portions in check. Choose wheat-free bread – such as spelt or rye – the flavour is much more pronounced and will provide a long-lasting energy boost.

- Salads are the perfect vehicle for upcycling yesterday's roasted vegetables. Simply toss them with chopped fresh herbs, cooked wild rice, a drizzle of extra virgin olive oil and a squeeze of lemon juice to make a nutritious and tasty meal.

- Baked potatoes or sweet potatoes are another versatile candidate for upcycling. They are given new life by simply topping with Lemony Creamed Spinach (see page 179) or Beetroot Tzatziki (see page 157).

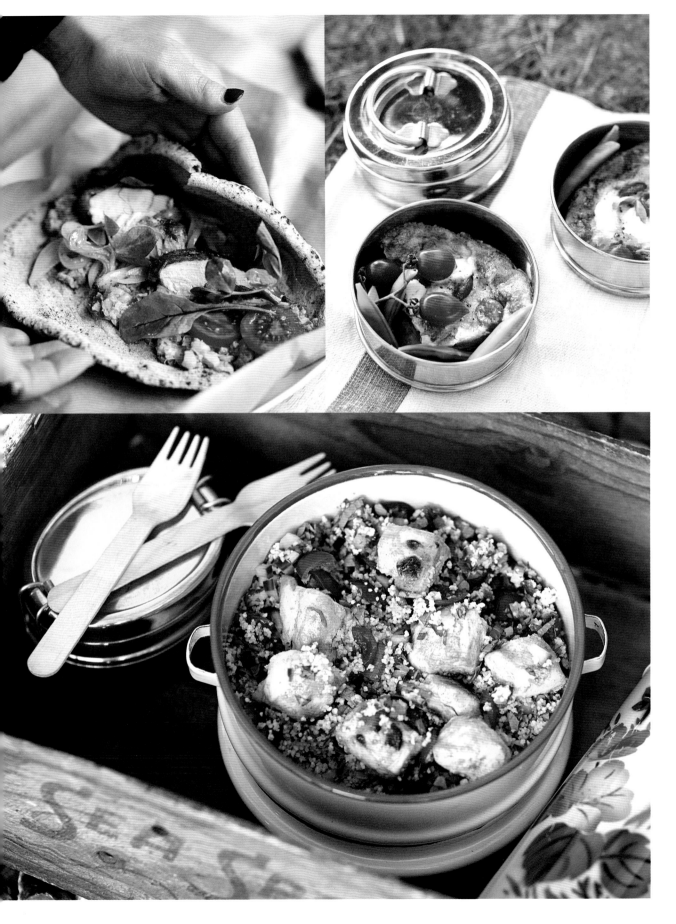

TECHNIQUES

I positively hate the thought of overcooked vegetables 'murdering your food', as I call it, is a sure-fire way to lose key nutrients. The most crucial starting point for every cook is to buy the best-quality produce you can afford. However, it is just as vital to know how to cook your ingredients in order to get the best out of them. Here, I've given a few techniques to make cooking quicker, easier and, more importantly, healthier.

Steaming

This is a healthy way to cook your food as it requires no oil. If you don't have a steamer, use an ordinary saucepan with a colander (or sieve) set over it, and place a large lid on top. Just make sure the boiling water isn't touching whatever you're steaming.

TIPS

- Keep an eye on the timing because you can quickly overcook food when steaming, turning it bland and mushy. You want vegetables to retain their colour, texture and bite, as well as their vitamins, minerals and other nutrients. (This is where steaming trumps boiling, a process which can too often leach minerals and vitamins out of the food.)

- Try steaming small portions of chicken or fish to get a delicate and gentle taste, a change from the harsh flavours that browning can sometimes produce.

- Steamed green vegetables will continue to cook after you have removed them from the steaming pan. If you are not serving them immediately, or are using them cold (e.g. in a salad), quickly run some cold water over them to halt the cooking process and preserve their colour.

- Sealing meat or fish in parchment paper or foil parcels to bake in the oven is a quick and low-fat method of steaming and all the delicious juices (and nutrients) are captured in the 'bag'. Avoid using foil if you are including any acidic ingredients such as tomatoes, because they react with the aluminium and won't taste very nice.

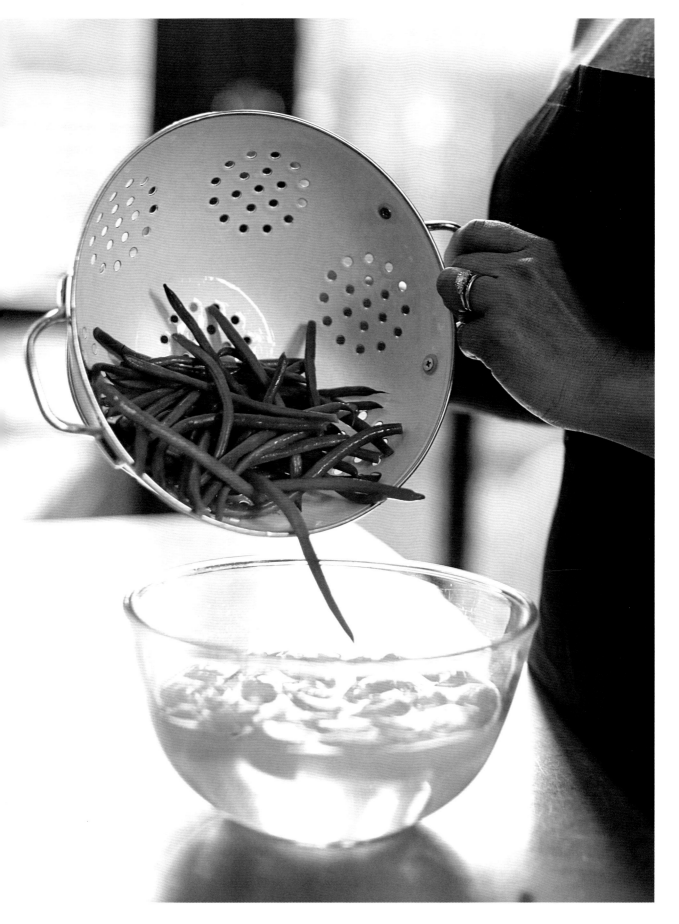

Blanching

This is a simple two-step process that involves plunging the ingredient into a pot of boiling water for a short time, and then transferring immediately into iced water to stop the cooking and preserve the food's colour and nutrients.

TIPS

- Make sure you have a bowl of iced water standing by before you start blanching your vegetables as you will need to work quickly.

- Don't overcook. A green vegetable that has turned brown or grey in colour has been overcooked and nutrients lost. Likewise, if the water you have cooked your greens in also turns green, then the vegetables have been in the pot for too long.

- To prevent avocados from turning brown in a salad, try blanching them whole (skin and all) for about a minute, and cooling them off in a bowl filled with iced water before serving. This will ensure that they stay green for longer and it also makes them easier to peel.

Grilling

Grilling (or broiling) is a quick and healthy way to brown meat or fish so that it is crisp on the outside but remains juicy and succulent on the inside. It is essential that the grill is preheated before you begin cooking.

TIPS

- Try to use tender cuts of meat no thicker than 4cm as they can easily burn on the outside before being cooked on the inside. Similarly, if you have marinated your meat or fish, be mindful of how easy it is for any oils in your marinade to catch fire.

- If you are worried that your food is being grilled too quickly on the outside, do not turn the heat down – rather move the food to a lower level.

Stir-frying

Stir-frying is an extremely fast cooking method; however, to do it efficiently, you need to have everything chopped and at the ready before you begin.

A wok is ideal for stir-frying – the rounded base means that the heat is highly concentrated in a small area, enabling you to brown meat and cook everything quickly. The roomy shape allows you to move the ingredients around to prevent scorching while the sloping sides bring them back to the heat centre. Having said all that, it won't be the end of the world if you use a large frying pan instead.

Very little oil is needed when you stir-fry, but because of the high heat involved it is best to use coconut, groundnut or rapeseed oil. Don't be tempted to use butter – it will just burn – and avoid extra virgin olive oil, as it also has a low smoking point.

TIPS

- Pre-chop all your vegetables. Slice them so that they are roughly the same size to ensure they cook evenly and at the same speed.

- Have any herbs and/or fresh chilli chopped, and sauces and seasoning standing by.

- Meat should be cubed and patted dry with kitchen paper to prevent it from stewing.

- Always start by browning the meat on a high temperature, with some oil. The very moment it starts to colour, you can then add the rest of the ingredients.

- Add any nuts, seeds or seasoning oils once the wok is off the heat. This keeps the good fats found in nuts and seeds or special oils from being ruined (exposure to high heat can transform them into bad fats).

- If you have the misfortune of burning anything, remove it, wipe the pan with some kitchen paper, and use clean oil to start over. You don't want to transfer the bitter charred taste to the rest of the dish.

breakfast

three ways with yoghurt 26

three ways with porridge 28

smoothies 30

breakfast cranachan 32

crêpes with cinnamon bananas 34

french toast with cinnamon & honey 36

cheese & corn muffins 38

garlic mushrooms on toast
with goat's curd 40

smoky baked eggs on rye 42

smoked salmon soufflé omelette 44

IT'S official: breakfast really is the most important meal of the day. Breakfast kick-starts the metabolism, which has, like an engine, been idle all night. It raises your glucose levels and sets up your energy stores for the day ahead.

It might be tempting to skip breakfast – and thereby cut your daily food consumption – but there are notable psychological and physiological downsides to doing this. In particular, you end up eating more, and badly, later in the day by way of compensation. I always find that if I miss breakfast, I'm guaranteed to hit a 'slump', which I try to fix by reaching for an instant solution – usually in a cookie jar or coffee cup.

Breakfast needn't be the same old toast or cereal dish thrown together morning after morning. To this end I've adapted many Pure Package favourites to make them even quicker and easier to prepare at home – such as Smoky Baked Eggs on Rye, or Smoked Salmon Soufflé Omelette, which are packed with vitamins, minerals and essential fats. Sweeter (but no less healthy) options include Strudel Porridge and Breakfast Cranachan, both of which are loaded with slow-burning carbs.

Hopefully the tempting recipes in this chapter will inspire you to start the day in the most delicious – and convenient – way.

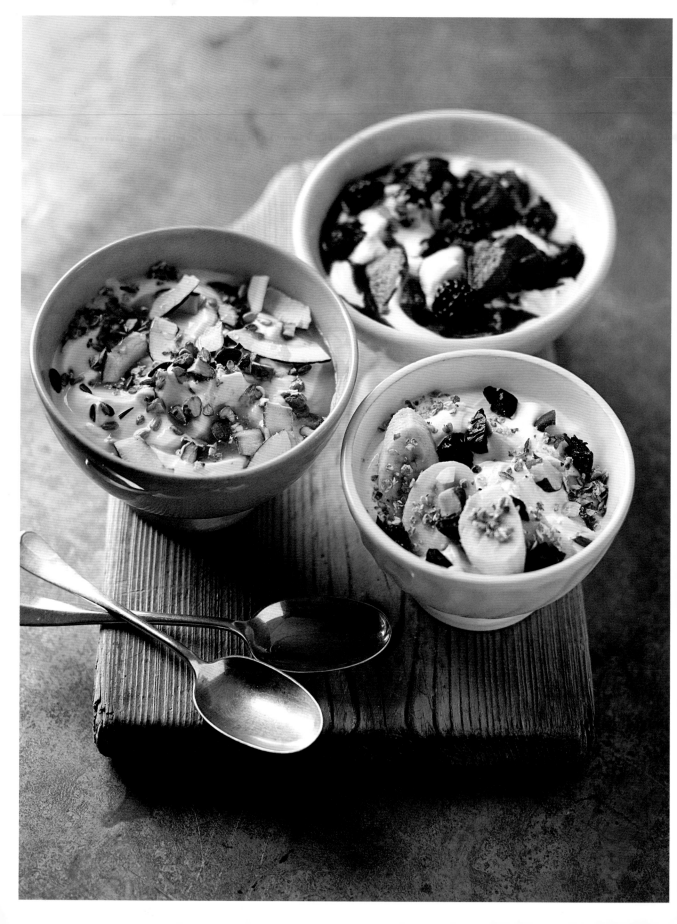

three ways with yoghurt

Serves: 2
Preparation time: 5–10 minutes
Vegetarian

What I have always loved about yoghurt is the myriad ways of dressing it up – there's very little that yoghurt doesn't combine well with. I prefer natural bio-yoghurt, made from cow's milk, topped with something crunchy, sweet or fruity. Here are three easy, nutritious and satisfying ways to get the most from your morning yoghurt.

with honeyed berries

1 tablespoon water
1 teaspoon honey
200g berries (strawberries, raspberries, or blackberries – or a mixture)

200g low-fat natural yoghurt
20g flaked almonds

To serve

Combine the water and honey in a non-stick saucepan over a medium heat. Add the berries and gently bring to the boil. Reduce the heat and leave to bubble for 4 minutes.

Spoon the yoghurt into 2 serving bowls and top with the warmed fruit, retaining the syrup.

Stir the yoghurt, fruit and almonds together. Spoon the warm syrup over the top.

with banana & brazil nuts

200g low-fat natural yoghurt

2 bananas, sliced
40g Brazil nuts, roughly chopped
20g flaked almonds
2 ready-to-eat prunes, stoned and roughly chopped

To serve

Divide the yoghurt between 2 serving bowls.

Top each bowl with equal amounts of chopped bananas, brazil nuts, flaked almonds and prunes.

Sprinkle over the yoghurt and fruit.

with seeds

2 tablespoons honey
1 tablespoon fresh orange juice
1 tablespoon fresh lime juice

200g low-fat natural yoghurt

1 tablespoon coconut flakes
2 tablespoons chopped unsalted pistachio nuts
1 tablespoon sunflower seeds
1 tablespoon pumpkin seeds

To serve
Small handful unsalted pistachio nuts, roughly chopped

Place the honey in a small pan with the orange and lime juice and warm gently over a low heat.

Divide the yoghurt between 2 serving bowls.

Top each bowl with equal amounts of coconut flakes, pistachio nuts and seeds.

Drizzle the warm honey mixture over each bowl and sprinkle with the toasted oats.

three ways with porridge

Serves: 2
Preparation time: 5–10 minutes
Vegetarian

Porridge is a winter breakfast staple in my house: it has the ability to help you start your day with a warm glow. Oats are an excellent source of slow-burning energy – they have a low GI (glycaemic index), meaning that the rate at which the sugar from the food is released into your bloodstream is slow. Choose thick, dehulled oats rather than rolled oats for making your porridge because they will keep you full for longer.

Toppings can be as simple or as involved as you like. From soft prunes with a drizzle of honey to more indulgent toppings like chopped banana, nuts and a trickle of chocolate sauce (see page 184), a bowl of porridge is the perfect canvas for creating a flavour-packed breakfast.

Here are three easy, nutritious ways to liven up your morning porridge, which are guaranteed to set you up for the day ahead.

strudel porridge

Preheat the grill to high.

60g jumbo porridge oats 200ml semi-skimmed milk 200ml cold water	Place the oats, milk and water in a non-stick pan.
1 apple, finely grated 30g raisins ½ teaspoon ground cinnamon	Add the apple, raisins and cinnamon, and stir well. Place the pan over a low heat, and leave to come slowly to the boil – this will take about 5 minutes. Stir occasionally to prevent clumping. Once it is bubbling, leave to simmer for another 2 minutes.
1 slice rye bread	Meanwhile, place the bread in a food processor or blender, and blend until you have fine breadcrumbs.
2 teaspoons honey	Transfer the breadcrumbs to a grill pan lined with foil and drizzle with honey. Grill for about 2 minutes, shaking the pan occasionally to ensure even toasting.
To serve	Divide the porridge between serving bowls, sprinkle with the toasted breadcrumbs and serve immediately.

peanut butter & banana porridge

60g jumbo porridge oats
200ml semi-skimmed milk
200ml cold water

Place the oats, milk and water in a non-stick pan. Place the pan over a low heat, and leave to come slowly to the boil – this will take about 5 minutes. Stir occasionally to prevent clumping. Once it is bubbling, leave to simmer for another 2 minutes.

2 tablespoons smooth unsalted peanut butter

Stir the peanut butter into the porridge, mixing well to blend.

Leave the porridge to warm through for a further minute, then spoon into 2 serving bowls.

1 banana, peeled and sliced

Divide the banana slices between the serving bowls.

To serve
Honey, to taste

Drizzle with honey and serve immediately.

cranberry & walnut porridge

80g jumbo porridge oats
200ml semi-skimmed milk
200ml cold water

Place the oats, milk and water in a non-stick pan. Place the pan over a low heat, and leave to come slowly to the boil – this will take about 5 minutes. Stir occasionally to prevent clumping. Once it is bubbling, leave to simmer for another 2 minutes.

3 tablespoons orange juice
1 tablespoon agave syrup

Meanwhile, place the orange juice and agave syrup into a small pan and bring to the boil over a low heat.

4 tablespoons fresh or frozen cranberries

Add the cranberries and return to the boil, then lower the heat and leave to simmer until the cranberries are tender but still holding their shape – about 5 minutes for frozen cranberries, and 8 minutes for fresh ones.

Gently spoon the cranberry sauce through the porridge, leaving a ripple effect.

To serve
Small handful walnuts, chopped

Divide the porridge between 2 serving bowls, top with the walnuts, and serve immediately.

smoothies

Serves: 2
Preparation time: 5–10 minutes
Vegetarian

Although I am a huge fan of breakfast, there are, inevitably, mornings when I don't have time to prepare and savour a proper meal. On days like this I turn to a home-made smoothie – which I refer to as 'breakfast in a glass', as they can give you everything a well-balanced, filling breakfast would, but are made in just minutes. Be as adventurous as you like with the fruit or vegetable combinations. Smoothies are the perfect vehicle for adding any food supplements you may require and for contributing to your five-a-day.

TIPS FOR MAKING REALLY GOOD SMOOTHIES

- Use an equal portion of fruit to liquid

- Use a maximum of three types of fruit, to retain the individual flavours

- Add vegetables – this is an easy and delicious way to eat the rainbow

- When using citrus fruit, squeeze the fruit first and use only the juice (the pith and pips will make the smoothie bitter as well as giving an unpleasant texture)

- Add frozen fruit. Bananas work particularly well – they're perfect for a slushy, frozen smoothie. Simply peel the banana, cut into chunks, and pop into a sealable freezer bag

- Prepare and drink smoothies fresh; if they are allowed to sit, they lose their nutritional goodness (you will notice that their colour fades)

I've suggested three recipes (see right), but I do hope that these will just be a starting point for you in creating your own smoothies.

The technique for creating them is the same: place all the ingredients in a blender, and process until it reaches the desired texture.

crunchy breakfast smoothie

INGREDIENTS

200ml semi-skimmed milk
3 tablespoons low-fat natural yoghurt
1 banana, peeled and cut into chunks
120g strawberries, hulled
1 tablespoon honey
80g granola or muesli

purple delight smoothie

INGREDIENTS

50ml fresh orange juice
50ml water
100ml low-fat yoghurt
50g raw cashew nuts
Large handful blackberries
Large handful blueberries
4 strawberries, hulled

green zing smoothie

INGREDIENTS

2 kiwis, peeled and cut into chunks
2 pears, peeled and cut into chunks
Flesh of ½ cantaloupe melon
100g baby spinach
50g unsalted pistachio nuts
200ml water
Juice of 2 limes

My husband is Scottish, and so naturally cranachan is a favourite in our house. While traditionally, cranachan is made with whisky, I created this lighter, alcohol-free version, with extra nuts and fruit, which is perfect for breakfast.

breakfast cranachan

Serves: 2
Preparation time: 10 minutes
Wheat free, Vegetarian

20g jumbo porridge oats

Place the oats in a non-stick frying pan and toast over a low heat, stirring regularly for about 3 minutes, or until they start to change colour. Transfer to a bowl to cool.

75g raspberries
75g blackberries

Place half of the each of the berries into a small mixing bowl and mash well with a fork.

100g low-fat natural yoghurt
100g half-fat crème fraîche

Add the yoghurt and crème fraîche, and stir to create a rippled effect.

2 tablespoons flaked almonds

Gently fold in the toasted oats, almonds and the whole berries. Save a handful of berries for decoration.

To serve
2 teaspoons honey

Divide the mixture between 2 serving glasses, and drizzle the honey on top to serve, and decorate with a few berries.

TIP Play around with a combination of any berries that are available, or you could double the amount of raspberries.

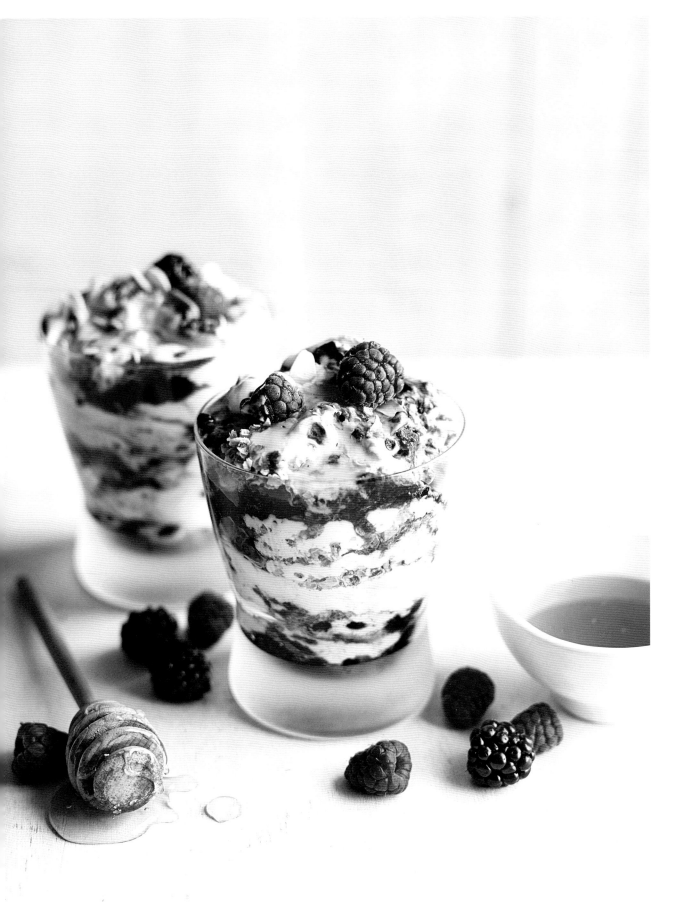

crêpes with cinnamon bananas

Serves: 4
Preparation time: 5 minutes
Cooking time: 20 minutes
Wheat free, Gluten free, Vegetarian
Preheat oven to 110°C/225°F/Gas mark ¼,
and place one large ovenproof plate inside

If you want to get your children interested in cooking, there's no easier way to start than with pancake batter – especially with this foolproof recipe.

150g gluten-free brown bread flour
2 eggs
450ml semi-skimmed milk

Sift the flour into a large mixing bowl. In a separate bowl, combine the eggs and milk, and pour slowly into the flour, whisking gently. When all of the egg mixture has been added, whisk more vigorously until you have a smooth pouring consistency. Transfer the mixture to a pouring jug.

2 ripe bananas, peeled and sliced
1 vanilla pod
2 teaspoons ground cinnamon

In a bowl, mash the bananas. Split the vanilla pod in half and using a sharp knife, scrape the seeds out. Add the cinnamon and vanilla seeds to the bananas.

1 teaspoon coconut oil, for frying

Heat the oil in a non-stick frying pan over a medium heat. Pour a small amount of the batter into the centre of the pan and swirl the mixture to the sides of the pan in a thin layer.

Leave the crêpe to cook, untouched, for about 2 minutes, then check that it is light brown underneath. If so, turn it and cook for a further 2 minutes on the other side. Transfer to the warmed plate, cover with a tea towel, and pop the plate back in the oven while you make the other crêpes.

Repeat the process, transferring each crêpe to the warm oven, until you have used up all the batter.

To serve
100g strawberries, hulled and quartered
Honey (optional)

Place a couple of tablespoons of the banana mixture in a line across the centre of each crêpe, add a few strawberries and a drizzle of honey (if using) then fold or roll up.

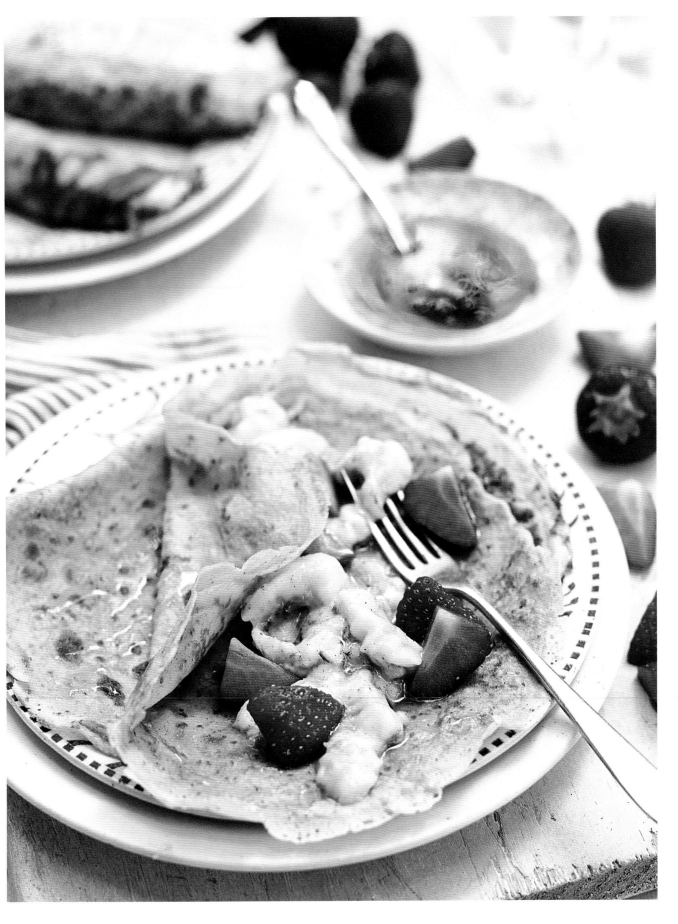

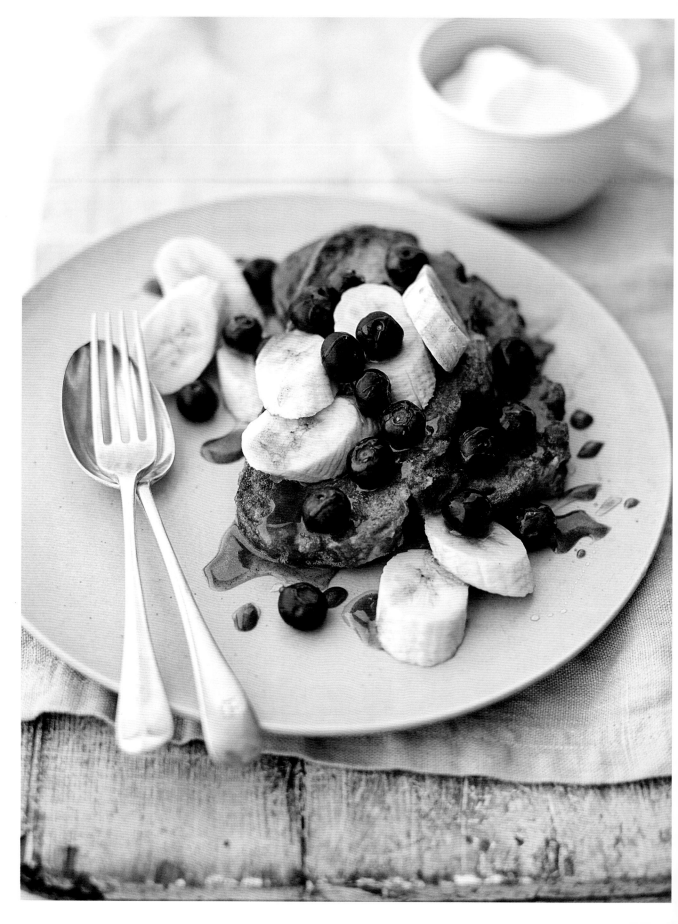

french toast with cinnamon & honey

Serves: 2
Preparation time: 10 minutes
Cooking time: 10 minutes
Vegetarian

This is my take on a classic. The difference being that instead of traditional white bread, I have used wholesome rye or spelt bread, which gives added texture and flavour to the finished dish.

2 medium free-range eggs

Beat the eggs in a bowl wide enough to hold both slices of bread.

2 slices rye or spelt bread

Cut the pieces of bread in half, and lay each slice in the egg.

Leave to soak for about a minute before turning over for another minute.

4 teaspoons honey
1 teaspoon ground cinnamon

Meanwhile, in a small bowl, mix together the honey and cinnamon.

Put the kettle on to boil and get a larger bowl. Put the small bowl inside the larger bowl and pour hot water into the large bowl, allowing the honey to warm through and become runny. Set aside.

1 teaspoon groundnut oil

Place the groundnut oil in a non-stick frying pan over a high heat. When hot, add the egg-soaked bread. Leave to cook for 2 minutes without moving, then flip over and cook on the other side for 1–2 minutes.

To serve
1 banana, sliced
100g blueberries
2 tablespoons half-fat crème fraîche

Divide the bread between the serving plates and drizzle with the cinnamon honey.

Top with banana slices and blueberries, dollop a tablespoon of crème fraîche on top, and eat immediately.

cheese & corn muffins

Makes:12
Preparation time: 15 minutes
Cooking time: 20–25 minutes
Wheat free, Vegetarian
Preheat oven to 190°C/375°F/Gas mark 5, and line
a 12-hole muffin tin with muffin cases

*Savoury muffins are a great way to
start the day – I think of them as being
halfway between toast and sweet muffins.
These are particularly mouthwatering
spread with cream cheese.*

50g brown rice flour
1 teaspoon bicarbonate of soda

Sieve the flour and bicarbonate of soda into a large
mixing bowl.

50g fine polenta
75g Parmesan, grated
2 spring onions, finely chopped
400g tin sweetcorn kernels, drained

Add the polenta, Parmesan, spring onions and half of the
sweetcorn kernels, and stir well to combine.

125ml buttermilk (alternatively use
100ml semi-skimmed milk mixed with
1 tablespoon half-fat soured cream,
white wine vinegar or lemon juice)

Place the buttermilk in a blender or food processor with the
remaining sweetcorn kernels and blend until quite smooth.

60ml sunflower oil
2 free-range eggs, beaten

Pour the milk mixture into a bowl and add the oil and eggs.
Mix well.

Pour the wet mixture into the dry ingredients and stir gently,
until just combined.

Spoon the batter into the muffin cases and place in the oven
for 20 minutes or until a skewer inserted into the centre comes
out clean.

To serve

Leave to cool for about 5 minutes, then serve while still warm.

TIP This recipe can also be used to make a nourishing and
delicious breakfast loaf. Pour the mixture into a 1lb loaf tin
and bake for 30 minutes, or until a skewer inserted comes out
clean. Slice and serve with scrambled eggs.

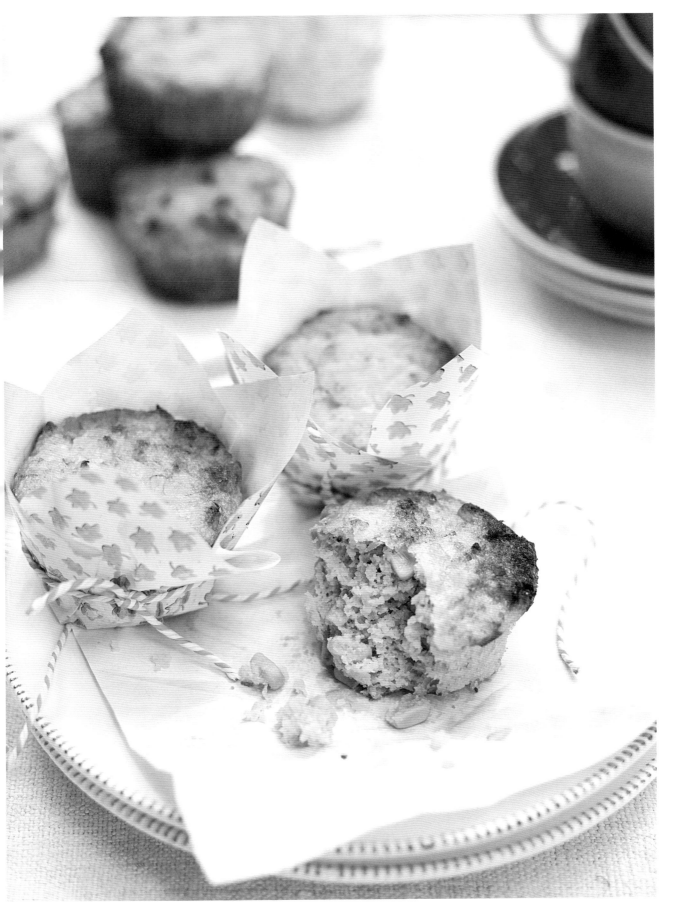

garlic mushrooms on toast with goat's curd

Serves: 2
Preparation time: 5 minutes
Cooking time: 15 minutes
Vegetarian

This dish is a childhood favourite, taking me back to the days of mushroom foraging near my family home. We often prepared them this way as the garlic and goat's curd are perfect partners for the earthy mushrooms.

20g unsalted butter

In a non-stick frying pan, heat the butter over a medium heat until foaming.

2 garlic cloves, crushed
1 shallot, finely chopped

Add the garlic and shallot, and sweat for a couple of minutes with the lid on, stirring occasionally, until soft.

300g chestnut mushrooms (or a mixture of wild mushrooms), sliced in half

Add the mushrooms and stir well, then leave to cook for 5–8 minutes until tender but still firm.

Freshly ground black pepper
Small handful flat-leaf parsley, finely chopped

Taste and season with black pepper, if needed, then stir in the parsley. Turn off the heat and cover the pan to keep the mixture warm.

2 slices spelt or rye bread
50g goat's curd, soft goat's cheese or half-fat cream cheese

Toast the bread, then spread each slice with the goat's curd.

To serve

Divide the toast between 2 plates, then spoon the mushroom mix on top.

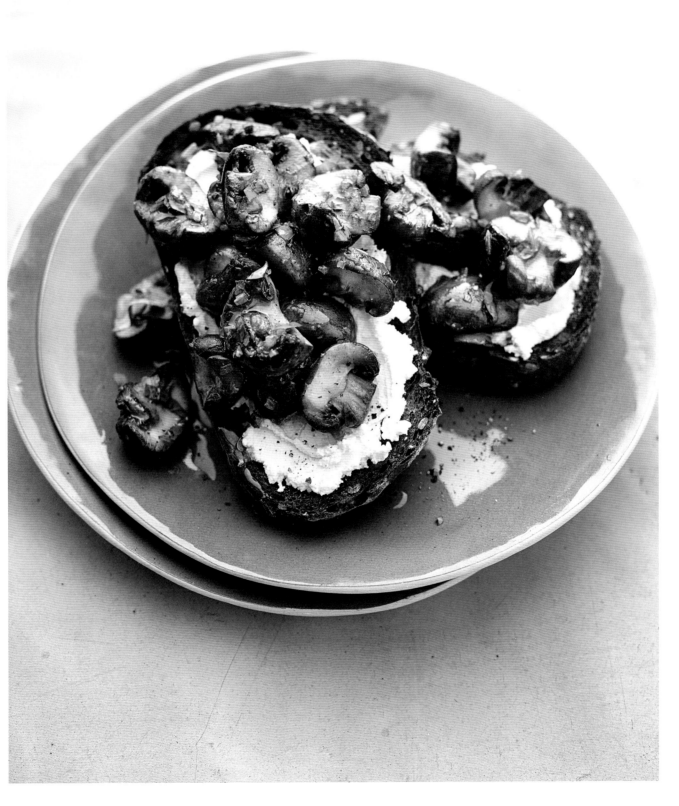

smoky baked eggs on rye

Inspired in part, by 'Turkish-style eggs' – poached eggs with paprika-flecked yoghurt – I've chosen to bake the eggs and have added iron-rich spinach and a portion of energy-filled rye bread.

Serves: 2
Preparation time: 10 minutes
Cooking time: 15 minutes
Dairy free, Vegetarian
Preheat oven to 220°C/425°F/Gas mark 7

1 teaspoon groundnut oil
1 garlic clove, crushed
1 teaspoon smoked paprika

Place the oil, garlic and paprika in a non-stick saucepan, and set over a medium heat.

200g baby spinach, washed

When the garlic starts to sizzle, add the spinach, stir well and cover. Leave to cook for 2–3 minutes with the lid on, until the spinach is wilted.

2 large free-range eggs

Divide the spinach and the garlicky oil between 2 lightly oiled ramekin dishes, then break an egg into each one.

2 tablespoons half-fat crème fraîche
Pinch smoked paprika

Spoon a tablespoon of crème fraîche over each egg, and sprinkle with a pinch of smoked paprika. Put in the oven for 15 minutes.

4 plum tomatoes

Put the tomatoes on the baking tray with the ramekins and roast for 15 minutes.

2 slices spelt or rye bread

Toast the spelt or rye bread. Use a knife to smash the cooked tomatoes on top of the toasted bread.

To serve

Serve the eggs in their ramekin dishes while still warm, with a slice of the tomato-topped toast accompanying each one.

TIP There's no limit to the number of ways you can serve baked eggs: choose any ingredients and pop them in the bottom of the ramekin dishes and top with an egg. Roasted red peppers, smoked salmon, and a few shavings of Parmesan all work well.

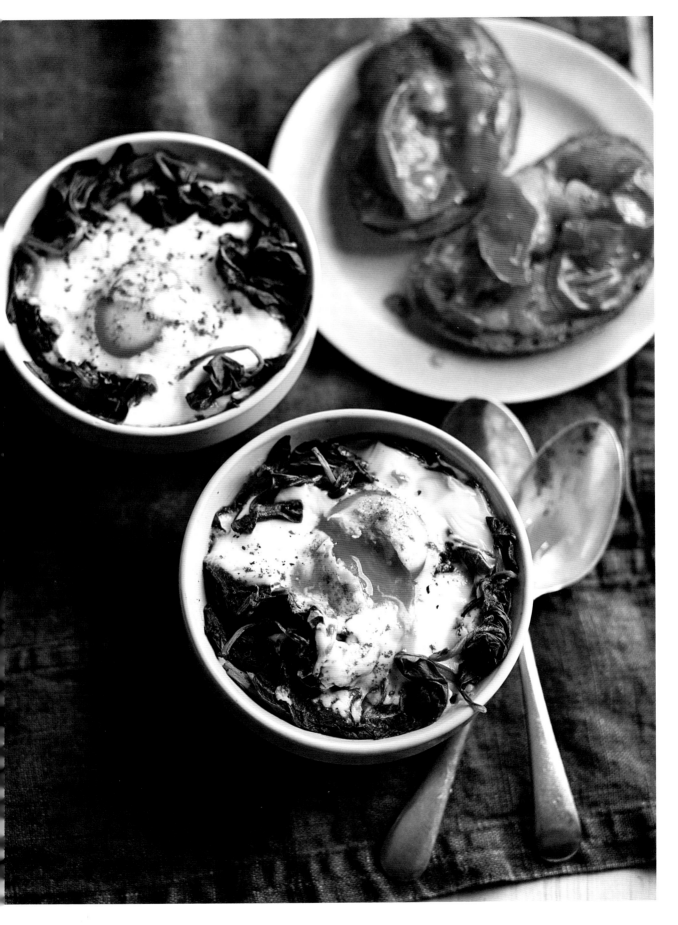

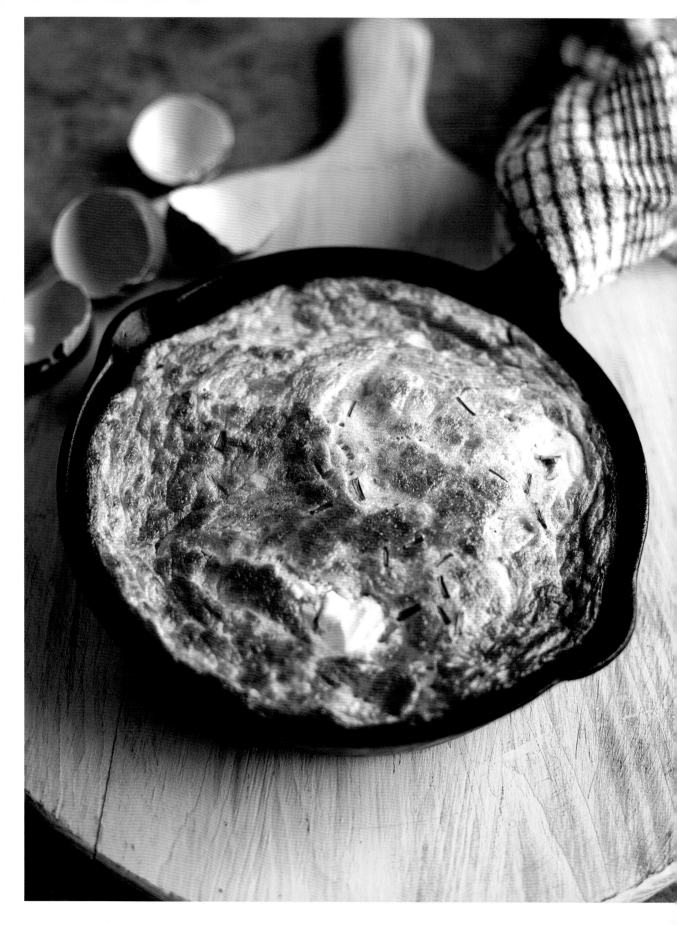

smoked salmon soufflé omelette

Serves: 2
Preparation time: 10 minutes
Cooking time: 15 minutes
Wheat free, Gluten free
Preheat grill to high

This is no ordinary omelette. It is stunning to look at and tastes so decadent – smoked salmon encased in fluffy eggs and oozing with cream cheese will make your mouth water!

1 tablespoon unsalted butter

Place the butter in a small pan over a medium heat.

1 tablespoon brown rice flour

When hot, add the rice flour, stirring constantly for 1 minute – it should resemble fine breadcrumbs.

100ml semi-skimmed milk
25g half-fat soured cream
25g low-fat crème fraîche

Mix the milk and soured cream until blended. Gradually add the milk mix to the pan and stir well, until it's slightly thick. Stir in the crème fraîche; the mixture should be nice and thick. Remove from the heat and pour into a large bowl.

3 large free-range eggs, separated

In a separate bowl, whisk the egg yolks until frothy, then add to the crème fraîche mix.

90g smoked salmon, finely sliced
1 heaped tablespoon chopped chives
40g half-fat cream cheese

Add the smoked salmon and chives to the egg-yolk mix. Stir well, then add the cream cheese in dollops, but don't mix it in.

In a separate bowl, whisk the egg whites to soft peaks, then gently fold them through the egg-yolk mixture.

1 teaspoon groundnut oil

Heat the oil in a non-stick frying pan over a medium heat, using kitchen paper to remove any excess oil from the pan.

Once the pan is nice and hot, pour in the egg mixture. Reduce the heat to low and cook for 2–3 minutes, until just set on the bottom. Do not stir.

Pop the frying pan under the grill for 4–5 minutes to brown the top.

To serve

Cut into slices and serve immediately.

TIP You can easily transform this into a vegetarian omelette by replacing the smoked salmon with three deseeded and diced plum tomatoes.

salads

GONE are the days when a salad consisted of limp lettuce leaves, drowning in an unctuous, lip-puckering sauce. Now the term 'salad' is becoming synonymous with fresh, vibrant eating; it's an opportunity to catch up on your five-a-day, while bringing together a variety of international flavours.

Salads are a fabulous way to explore interesting combinations of flavours, textures and even temperatures. They can be warm and comforting or zingy, fresh and summery. You can be as indulgent as you like with luxurious ingredients such as smoked salmon and caviar, or experiment by using exotic fruits as centrepieces.

At The Pure Package we work hard to ensure that our salads excite both the eye and the palate – but also that they are substantial, always comprising a well-balanced meal. This is why you will find roasted vegetables – with all the goodness of their vitamins and fibre sealed in – taking centre-stage in one salad, while protein-rich pulses or omega-oil-dense fish feature in others. To these I've added nuts full of essential fats, creamy avocados, citrus-infused dressings – and even the occasional crunchy fruit.

In this chapter you will discover some of our most popular creations, as well as many new ones. All of them are quick and easy – and bursting with goodness.

greek superfood salad

Serves: 2
Preparation time: 15 minutes
Cooking time: 15 minutes
Wheat free, Vegetarian
Preheat grill to high

Our superfood salad is so-called because it's packed with nutrients and vitamin-rich ingredients. The addition of olives gives this salad a Mediterranean twist that is certain to bring some sunshine to your day.

40g quinoa, rinsed

Cook the quinoa in boiling water for about 12 minutes – or according to the packet instructions. Drain and rinse under cold water.

125g halloumi, cut into thin slices
8 black olives, pitted and halved

Meanwhile, soak the halloumi slices and olives in water for 10 minutes, to remove any excess salt.

4 tablespoons barley couscous
120ml vegetable stock, boiling
1 teaspoon extra virgin olive oil

While the cheese and olives are soaking, place the couscous in a deep bowl and cover with the vegetable stock. Stir in the olive oil and cover the bowl with cling film. Set aside for 5 minutes.

8 cherry tomatoes, halved
¼ cucumber, peeled and cut into dice
Small handful flat-leaf parsley, roughly chopped
Handful fresh mint, roughly chopped

In a bowl mix the tomatoes, cucumber, drained olives, parsley and mint. Add the quinoa and couscous and stir to combine.

1 tablespoon extra virgin olive oil
1 tablespoon lemon juice

Whisk together the olive oil and lemon juice, and add half to the vegetables and grains.

Drain the halloumi, pat dry, and place under the hot grill for 3 minutes on each side, until browned and crispy (alternatively, dry-fry them in a small non-stick frying pan for a minute on each side over a high heat).

To serve
Freshly ground black pepper

Divide the couscous mixture between serving plates, along with the halloumi slices and drizzle with the remaining dressing. Season with black pepper and serve.

TIP If you can't find halloumi, use chunks of ungrilled feta instead and soak in the same way before adding to the salad.

UPCYCLE If you make too much salad you can easily transform it into a nutritious lunch the next day. Simply spread wholemeal pitta bread with some hummus and fill with Greek Superfood Salad.

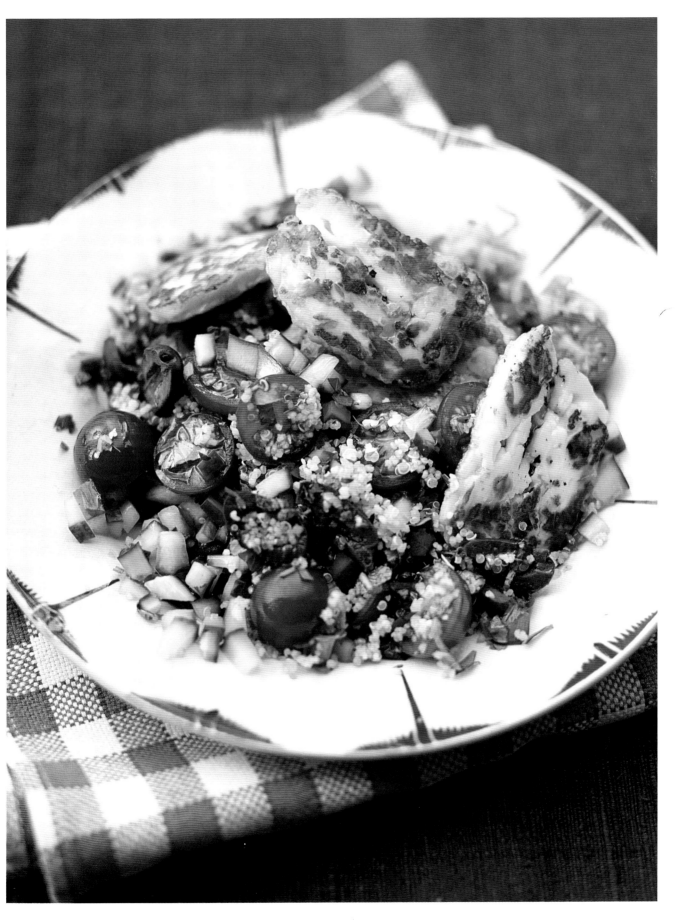

three-bean salad with quail's eggs

Serves: 2
Preparation time: 10 minutes
Cooking time: 15 minutes
Wheat free, Gluten free, Dairy free, Vegetarian

For too long green beans have had an unfair reputation as 'soggy vegetables'. This delightful, crunchy salad aims to reverse that, tossing them with other beans in a zingy, lively dressing. Just make sure you drop the beans in iced water to preserve their crunch.

150g baby potatoes, scrubbed and halved

Place the potatoes in a pan of boiling water and simmer until cooked through – about 10 minutes. Drain and leave to cool by running under cold water.

140g fine green beans, topped and tailed (have a bowl of iced water at the ready)

Bring a separate pan of water to the boil and blanch the green beans: plunge then into the boiling water for 90 seconds, then remove from the pan with a slotted spoon and dunk into a bowl of iced water. Drain and place in a large salad bowl.

6 fresh quail's eggs

Carefully place the quail's eggs in the pan of hot water that you used to cook the beans, and leave to simmer for 2 minutes. Remove and place in a bowl of cold water for a few moments. Then peel them and cut in half. Set aside.

2 tablespoons lemon juice
½ green chilli, deseeded and finely chopped
1 spring onion, finely chopped
1 tablespoon cold water

Meanwhile, make the dressing. Mix the lemon juice, green chilli, spring onion and water. Set aside.

2 spring onions, finely chopped
100g tin cannellini beans, drained and rinsed
100g tin butter beans, drained and rinsed
Small handful fresh chives, finely chopped
Small handful fresh parsley, finely chopped
Small handful fresh mint, finely chopped

Add the spring onions, cannellini beans, butter beans, chives, parsley and mint to the bowl containing the green beans. Stir well.

Toss with the baby potatoes and the dressing.

To serve
Large handful watercress, large stalks removed

Divide the watercress leaves between serving plates, top with the dressed potatoes and beans, then scatter over the quail's eggs.

TIP The miniature size of quail's eggs complements the beans perfectly, but you can easily use two hardboiled hen's eggs instead and serve them quartered.

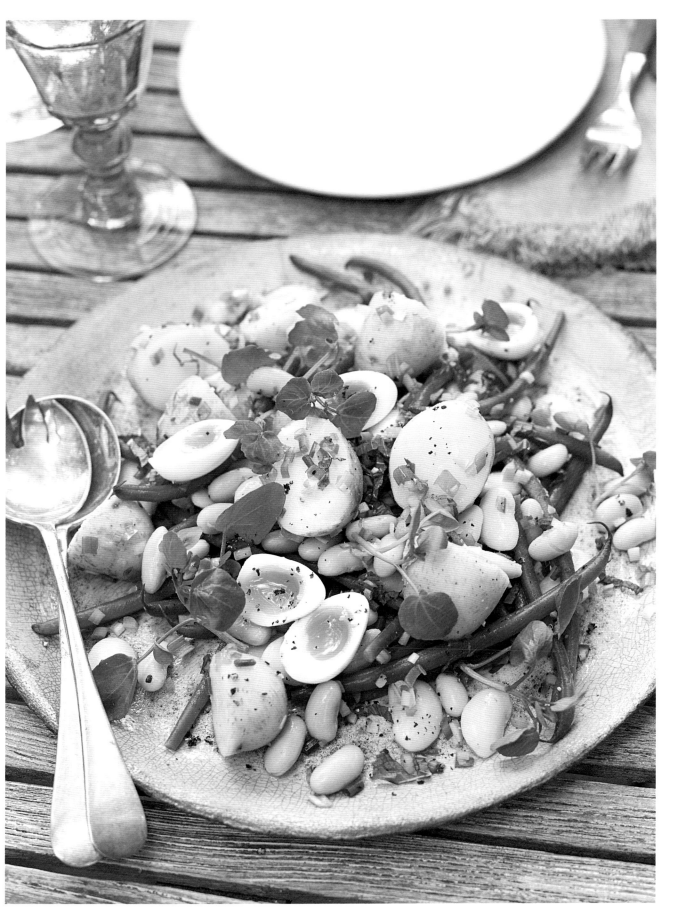

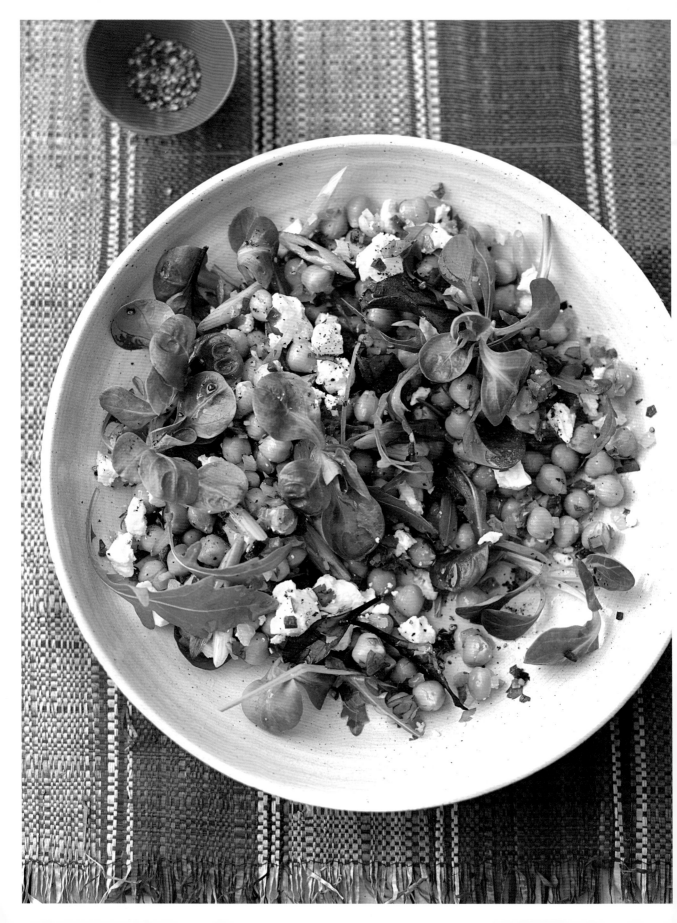

chickpea, chilli & feta salad

My friend Gaby came up with this recipe, perfectly balancing the chilli and garlic heat with the creaminess of the feta and the nutty bite of the chickpeas.

Serves: 2
Preparation time: 10 minutes
Cooking time: 10 minutes
Wheat free, Gluten free, Vegetarian

1 tablespoon olive oil
1 large red chilli, deseeded and finely chopped
3 garlic cloves, peeled and finely chopped
1 red onion, peeled and finely chopped

40ml cider or white wine vinegar

400g tin chickpeas, drained and rinsed
80g feta cheese, crumbled
2 tablespoons extra virgin olive oil
2 spring onions, finely sliced
Small handful fresh coriander, finely chopped
Small handful flat-leaf parsley, finely chopped
Freshly ground black pepper

To serve
2 handfuls baby leaves (such as rocket, lamb's lettuce, or a mixed variety)

In a small non-stick pan, heat the oil, chilli, garlic and onion over a medium heat. Sweat for 3–5 minutes (or until the garlic starts to brown), stirring constantly to prevent sticking.

Add the vinegar and leave to boil rapidly, until the liquid has almost completely evaporated – about 3–5 minutes.

In a bowl mix the chickpeas, chilli and onion mix, feta cheese, olive oil, spring onions, coriander and parsley, and stir well. Season to taste with black pepper.

Divide the chickpea mix between serving plates and top with the mixed leaves. Serve immediately.

UPCYCLE Toss any leftover salad with couscous and lemon zest for a quick and easy meal for one.

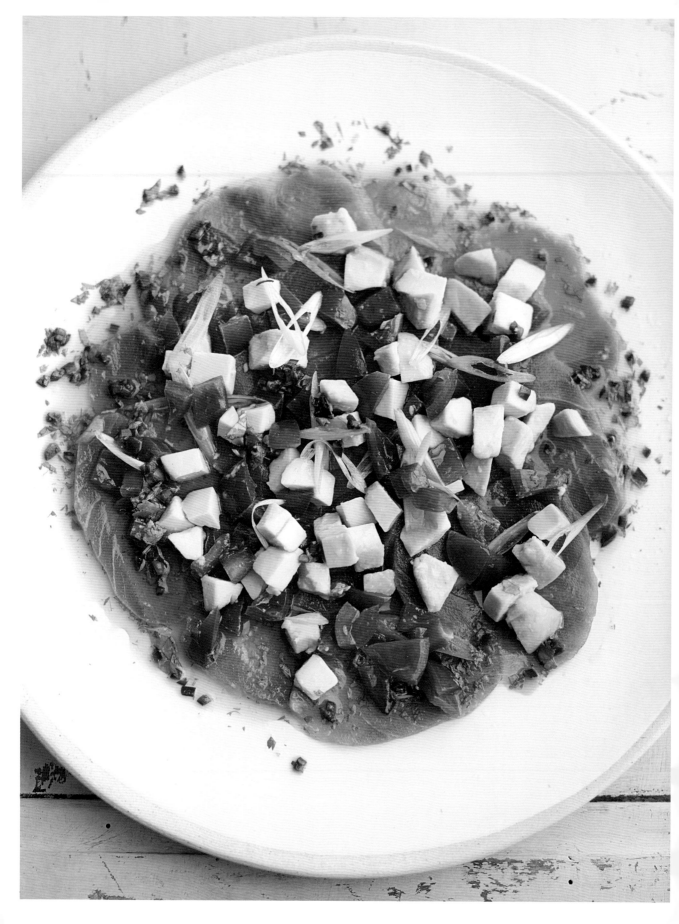

In this salad, fish is 'cooked' in citrus juices, infusing it with a dose of vitamin C. Use the freshest fish you can find and slice it as thinly as possible. I've used tuna for this recipe, but use any firm fish available such as sea bass or kingfish.

ceviche

Serves 2
Preparation time: 25 minutes
Wheat free, Gluten free, Dairy free

200g super-fresh tuna fillets, skinned and boned

Juice of 2 limes
1 red chilli, deseeded and finely chopped
2 tablespoons finely chopped coriander

1 avocado, peeled, stone removed, and chopped into small dice
2 plum tomatoes, deseeded and diced
1 spring onion, finely sliced
1 tablespoon olive oil

To serve
Freshly ground black pepper

Slice the fish into very thin – almost see-through – slices.

In a small bowl, mix the lime juice, chilli and coriander.

Place the fish in a wide glass or earthenware dish, so that the slices are barely overlapping, and spoon over the lime-juice mix, ensuring that every piece of fish is covered. Place kitchen paper over the dish and set aside for 10 minutes.

Meanwhile, place the avocado, tomatoes and spring onion in a salad bowl, add the olive oil, and toss.

Scatter the salad over the fish slices and spoon over the lime dressing. Season with black pepper and serve immediately.

TIP You can always substitute lemon juice for lime juice, or use a mixture of the two.

UPCYCLE Fill a corn wrap or flatbread with any leftover ceviche along with baby spinach leaves and top with soured cream for a quick and delicious lunch.

prawn cocktail with virgin mary sauce

This classic eighties starter makes a wonderful protein-packed lunch. We've added our own twist, in the form of puréed avocado, to ensure you get some great essential fats.

Serves: 2
Preparation time: 15 minutes
Cooking time: 3 minutes
Wheat free

1 little gem lettuce, shredded
4 cherry tomatoes, halved
¼ cucumber, diced
9 asparagus tips, finely sliced
5 radishes, finely sliced

½ avocado, stone removed
Small handful fresh coriander, finely chopped
Good squeeze lemon juice

50ml spiced tomato juice (if unavailable, add 1 teaspoon Tabasco to 50ml tomato juice)
2 tablespoons half-fat crème fraîche
½ teaspoon Worcestershire sauce
½ teaspoon horseradish paste

To serve
160g large cooked prawns
Lemon wedges
2 slices rye bread (optional)

Mix the lettuce, tomatoes and cucumber in a bowl. Layer the asparagus and radish on top of the lettuce mix.

Spoon the avocado flesh into another bowl, and mash until smooth. Add the coriander and lemon juice and mix well until combined.

In another bowl, mix the spiced tomato juice, crème fraîche, Worcestershire sauce and horseradish. Stir well to mix.

Put the salad mix into serving glasses and top with the avocado purée. Place the prawns on top and finish with the tomato sauce.

Serve with lemon wedges along with a couple slices of rye bread (if using).

UPCYCLE This makes a very special open sandwich. Chop the prawns into bite-sized pieces and mix through the salad vegetables with the tomato dressing. Spread the avocado purée onto a slice of rye bread and top with the prawn mix.

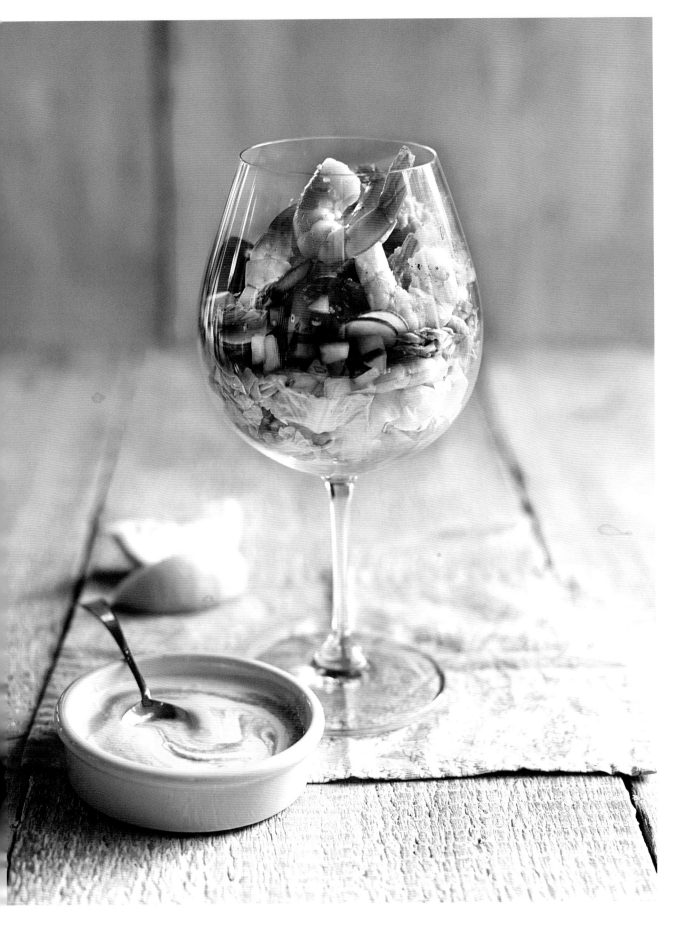

smoked mackerel & potato salad

Serves: 2
Preparation time: 15 minutes
Cooking time: 15 minutes
Wheat free, Gluten free

Smoked mackerel is the ultimate convenience food: already cooked for you, and packed full of essential fats. I've paired it with baby potatoes so that the protein of the fish is balanced by a slow-burning carbohydrate.

8 baby or new potatoes, halved

Cook the potatoes in a pan of boiling water for 10–15 minutes until tender. Drain and cool by running under cold water.

5 tablespoons low-fat natural yoghurt
Juice of 1 lemon
Freshly ground black pepper
Small handful flat-leaf parsley, finely chopped

Mix the yoghurt with the lemon juice and season to taste with black pepper. Add the parsley and stir well. Set aside for the flavours to infuse.

100g lamb's lettuce or baby spinach leaves
½ small cucumber, peeled and sliced
4 baby plum or cherry tomatoes, halved

Place the salad leaves, cucumber and tomatoes on a large serving plate. Top with the cooled potatoes.

2 small smoked mackerel fillets

Remove the skin from the mackerel, flake the fillets into bite-sized pieces, and scatter on top of the salad.

To serve
Freshly ground black pepper

Spoon over the yoghurt dressing, and toss together before serving. Finish with a final twist of black pepper.

UPCYCLE For a delicious way to upcycle mackerel fillets, mash the flaked fish thoroughly with the dressing ingredients to make a chunky pâté, and serve on toasted rye bread.

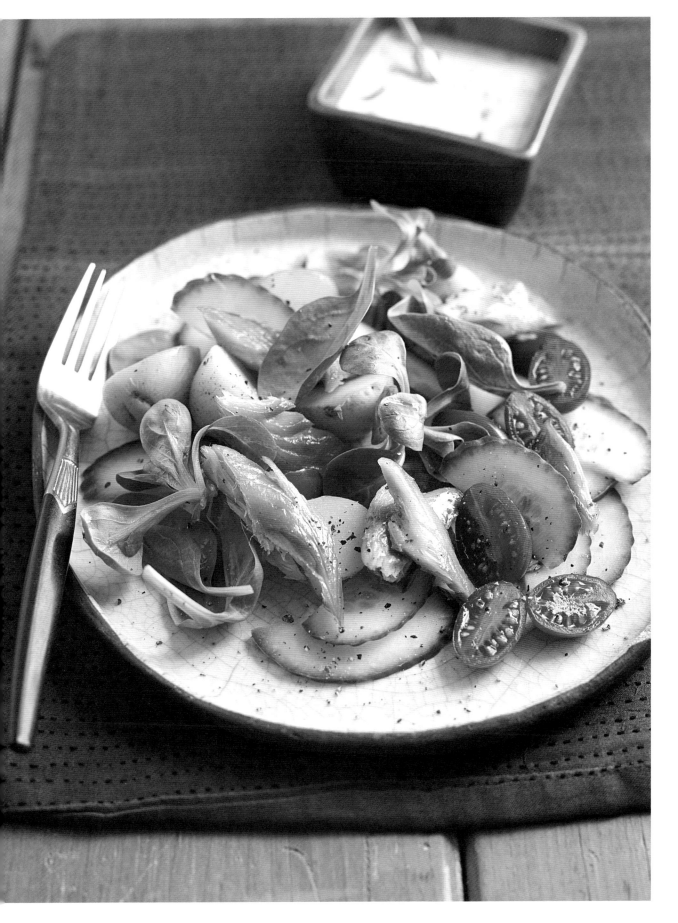

cajun chicken with black-eyed bean salsa

Serves 2
Preparation time: 25 minutes
Cooking time: 10 minutes
Wheat free, Gluten free

In this salad, chicken is marinated in aromatic spices, giving it a wonderful depth of flavour, offset by the smooth texture of the beans and the crunch of corn and peppers.

For the Cajun spice mix
2 teaspoons olive oil
½ teaspoon paprika
¼ teaspoon dried oregano
¼ teaspoon cayenne pepper
¼ teaspoon dried thyme
1 garlic clove, finely chopped

First, make the Cajun spice mix. In a large bowl, mix together the olive oil, paprika, oregano, cayenne pepper, thyme and garlic.

2 small free-range chicken breasts, skin removed, cut into strips

Place the chicken pieces in the bowl with the spices and mix thoroughly, so that the chicken is completely covered. Set aside to marinate for 10 minutes.

200g tin black-eyed beans, drained
2 tomatoes, deseeded and cut into small dice
80g tin sweetcorn kernels, drained
2 spring onions, finely chopped
15g sun-dried tomatoes, diced
Zest and juice of 1 lime
Small handful fresh coriander, finely chopped

Next make the salsa. In a large bowl, mix the beans, tomatoes, sweetcorn, spring onions, sun-dried tomatoes, lime zest and juice, and coriander. Stir well and put to one side.

3 tablespoons half-fat soured cream
1 jalapeño pepper (from a jar), finely diced
Juice of 1 lime

In a separate bowl, mix together the soured cream and jalapeño pepper. Add the lime juice and stir well.

2 teaspoons groundnut oil

Put the oil in a non-stick pan over a medium heat, then add the chicken. Leave to cook for 2–3 minutes without moving, then flip and cook on the other side for a further 2–3 minutes, or until cooked through.

To serve

Place the salsa mixture on a large serving plate, top with the warm chicken, and drizzle over the dressing.

UPCYCLE This is delicious topping for baked sweet potatoes. Slice up the chicken and stir through the salsa then stir through a dollop of soured cream.

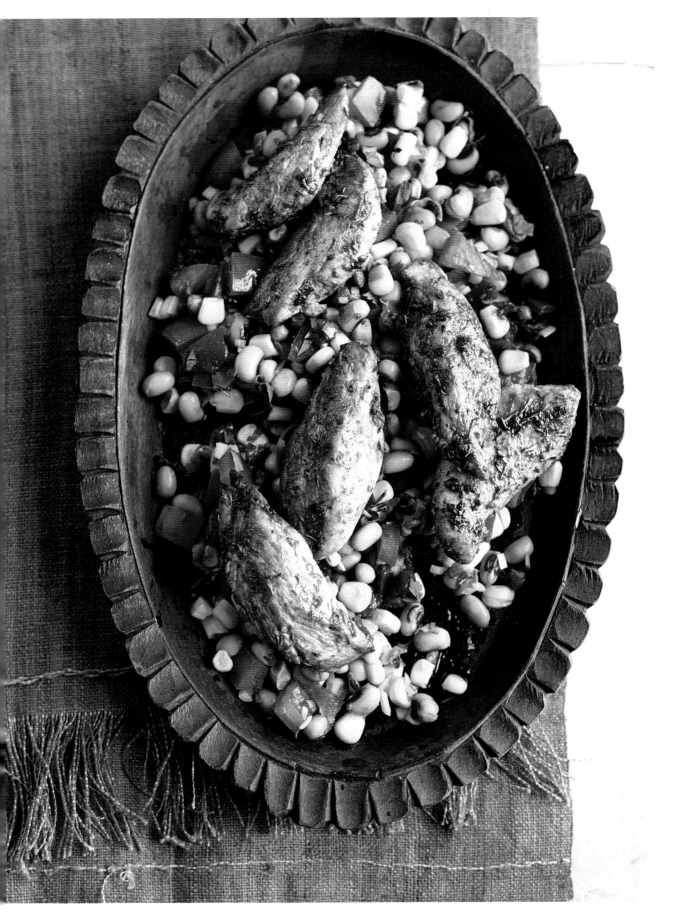

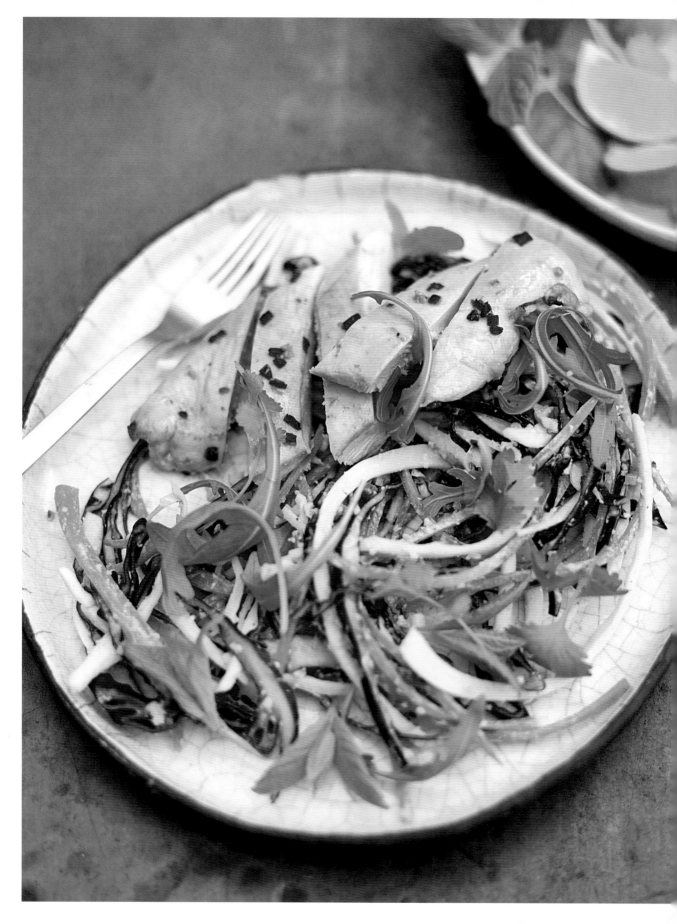

vietnamese chicken with ginger & peanut coleslaw

Warm, succulent chicken tossed with fresh crunchy vegetables are brought together by a vibrant zingy dressing in this salad.

Serves: 2
Preparation time: 15 minutes
Cooking time: 15 minutes
Wheat free, Gluten free, Dairy free
Preheat oven to 200°C/400°F/Gas mark 6, and place a non-stick baking tray inside

½ red chilli, deseeded and finely chopped
1 garlic clove, crushed
1 tablespoon rice vinegar
1 tablespoon lime juice
1 tablespoon Thai fish sauce
2 small free-range chicken breasts, skin removed

1 red chilli, deseeded and roughly chopped
3cm piece fresh ginger, peeled and roughly chopped
25g raw peanuts, roughly chopped
2 tablespoons smooth peanut butter
200ml half-fat coconut milk
Juice of ½ lime

2 carrots, peeled and finely sliced into strips
¼ head of red cabbage, finely sliced into strips
¼ head of white cabbage, finely sliced into strips

To serve
Small handful fresh mint leaves, roughly chopped
Small handful fresh coriander leaves, roughly chopped
Handful rocket leaves

Mix the chilli, garlic, rice vinegar, lime juice and fish sauce together into a thick paste. Rub into the chicken breasts.

Place the chicken on the hot baking tray and roast in the oven for 15 minutes, checking that the chicken is cooked through.

Meanwhile, make the dressing by placing the chilli, ginger, peanuts, peanut butter, coconut milk and lime juice in a food processor and blend until smooth.

Next, make the coleslaw by placing the carrots and red and white cabbage into a large serving bowl. Mix with the dressing, reserving 2 tablespoons. Divide the coleslaw between 2 serving plates.

Slice the chicken at an angle into nice bite-sized pieces.

Mix together the herbs and rocket leaves and place on top of the coleslaw.

Place the warm chicken on top of the coleslaw, then spoon the remaining dressing and cooking juices over the chicken.

TIP If you want to use ready cooked chicken, make extra dressing and mix it with the sliced chicken before serving.

UPCYCLE For a healthy and substantial lunch or supper, mix any leftover portions of this salad with a helping of cooked and drained rice noodles and serve either hot or cold.

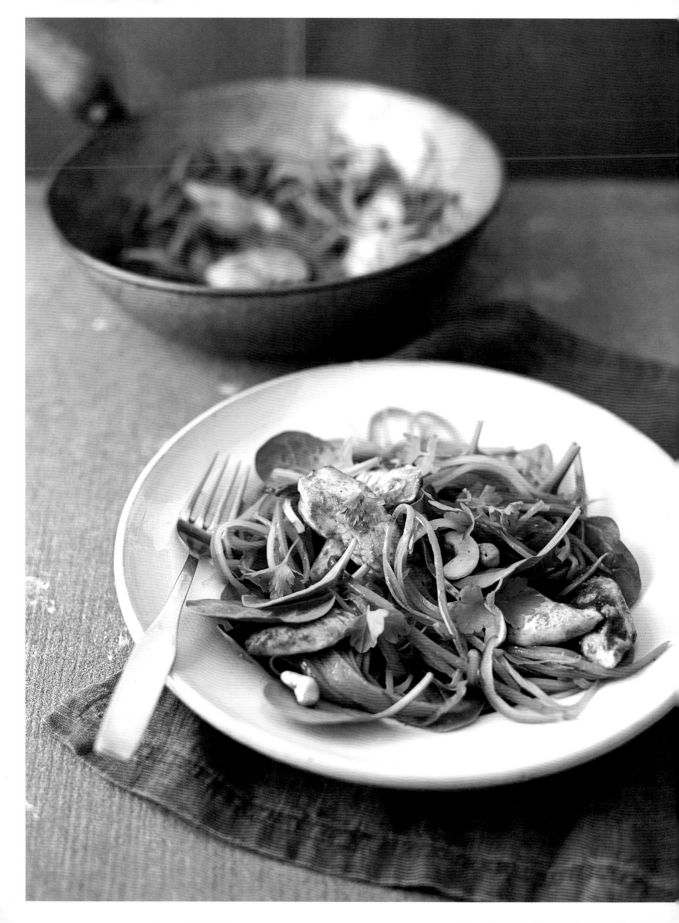

hot honeyed chicken salad

I love warm salads. This all-time favourite was inspired by my foodie friend Gaby. It is sweet enough to entice children, yet savoury and deliciously crunchy enough for adults. A sure winner!

Serves: 2
Preparation time: 10 minutes
Cooking time: 10 minutes
Wheat free, Gluten free, Dairy free

2 teaspoons sesame oil
2 small free-range chicken breasts, skin removed, cut into thin strips

2 carrots, peeled and cut into thin strips
2 celery stalks, cut into thin strips
1 red onion, finely sliced

1 tablespoon tomato purée
1 tablespoon honey
¼ teaspoon curry powder

2 handfuls baby spinach

To serve
Small handful flat-leaf parsley
20g unsalted cashew nuts

Heat the oil in a wok or heavy-based frying pan over a medium–high heat. Add the chicken, and cook for about 2 minutes.

Add the carrots, celery and onion to the pan, cover with the lid or some foil and cook for a further 5 minutes until the onion is soft and the chicken is cooked.

Meanwhile, make the dressing. In a small bowl combine the tomato purée, honey and curry powder, and stir. Add to the pan and mix through for a couple of minutes.

Place the baby spinach into serving bowls. Top with the chicken and vegetables hot from the pan.

Garnish with the parsley and cashew nuts.

TIP This recipe works well with leftover cooked chicken also – simply shred the chicken and add to the vegetable mix before you add the dressing. When heated through, add the dressing, parsley and nuts.

UPCYCLE Once cooled, the flavours of the salad develop further, making it a perfect filling for a soft corn tortilla wrap.

very pink salad

A Sunday roast of beef with horseradish is a match made in heaven. When I don't have the time – or inclination – to make a roast but crave the flavours, this salad provides a taste of all the component parts but with the added peppery crunch of watercress.

Serves: 2
Preparation time: 20 minutes
Cooking time: 3 minutes
Wheat free, Gluten free

160g lean fillet of beef

Take the fillet of beef out of the fridge and allow it to come to room temperature 20 minutes before cooking.

1 tablespoon groundnut oil

Heat the oil in a medium non-stick frying pan, then fry the beef over a high heat for 1 minute on each side. Remove from the pan and leave to rest.

1 teaspoon fresh horseradish paste
2 tablespoons low-fat natural yoghurt
1 tablespoon olive oil
Juice of 1 lemon
1 teaspoon Dijon mustard
4 small beetroot, ready cooked, chopped into bite-sized pieces

Next make the dressing. Mix together the horseradish, yoghurt, olive oil, lemon juice and mustard, stirring well to combine. Add the beetroot and mix until the dressing turns pink.

To serve
3 large handfuls watercress, large stems removed
2 spring onions, chopped
Freshly ground black pepper
2 slices rye bread (optional)

Slice the rested beef thinly and arrange on serving plates. Remove the beetroot pieces from the dressing and place on top. Scatter the watercress and spring onions over and season with black pepper. Serve alongside rye bread, if you like.

UPCYCLE This salad is particularly good as an open sandwich filling, topped with sliced radishes.

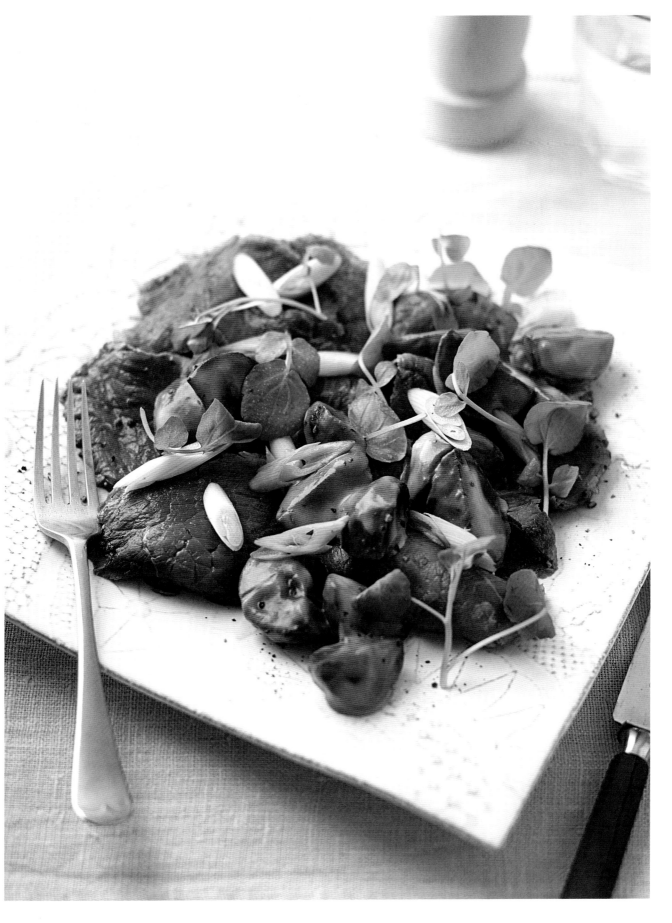

soups

SOUPS

are a clever way of consuming more vegetables, while being some of the simplest and quickest dishes to prepare. With very little effort you can create a cheap, nutritious meal, packed full of goodness for you and your family. It's also one of the best ways to help you increase your daily intake of vitamins, minerals and essential fats, while at the same time filling you with wonderful energy-releasing carbs and cell-repairing proteins.

The process of making soup – often blending vegetables with their cooking water – ensures that nutrients which might otherwise be lost from raw ingredients during cooking remain in the broth. Vegetables that might be difficult to consume or digest raw (such as sweet potatoes, which are rich in vitamin E, or fibre-dense celeriac) are made more palatable and digestible, thus enabling us to eat them in greater quantities.

For a balanced meal that will sustain you for longer, accompany your chosen soup with a portion of protein such as cream cheese on rye crackers. Good-quality stock will be your go-to ingredient for these recipes and for convenience, buy quality ready-made stock at the supermarket.

Once you've tried the recipes in this chapter, you'll be amazed at how easy they are to prepare, and just how good they taste.

tomato & red pepper soup

Serves: 2
Preparation time: 10 minutes
Cooking time: 30 minutes
Wheat free, Gluten free, Dairy free, Vegetarian

Charred peppers give this tomato soup a smokiness that goes well with the hint of chilli. The vibrant colour will really make you feel like you're eating he rainbow – or at least part of it!

1 tablespoon groundnut oil
1 small onion, very finely chopped

Heat the oil in a large saucepan over a medium heat. Add the onion and sweat for 3 minutes.

4 medium tomatoes, finely chopped
1 red pepper, deseeded and finely chopped
1 small garlic clove, peeled and finely chopped
½ red chilli, deseeded and finely chopped
Small handful basil leaves, roughly chopped

Add the tomatoes, pepper, garlic, chilli and basil, and stir to mix. Cover and leave to sweat for 5 minutes, stirring occasionally to prevent sticking.

2 tablespoons tomato purée
1 tablespoon red wine vinegar
500ml vegetable stock

Add the tomato purée, vinegar and vegetable stock. Bring to the boil, then reduce the heat and simmer for 20 minutes.

1 red pepper, stalks removed, deseeded and cut into thick slices

Meanwhile, prepare the additional pepper. Grill the slices under a hot grill, turning occasionally, until blackened. (Alternatively, hold the whole pepper over a gas flame, turning constantly, until completely charred.) Place the blackened slices in a plastic bag and hold closed, shaking, for a couple of minutes. When cool enough to handle, peel off the charred skin and dice the flesh.

1 tomato

Make a small cross incision at the base of the tomato, then drop into a bowl of boiled water. Leave for 1–2 minutes before removing with a slotted spoon. The skin should have started to peel, making it easy to slip the skin away from the flesh. Quarter the skinned tomato and squeeze it firmly over a bowl to release the seeds. Chop the tomato flesh and mix with the diced pepper. Set aside.

Blend the soup until smooth, using a hand-held blender or by transferring to a food processor.

To serve
2 teaspoons Basil Pesto (see page 96)
Parmesan cheese, grated (optional)

Ladle the soup into warmed bowls, garnishing each serving with a teaspoon of pesto, Parmesan (if using) and some roasted pepper and tomato mix.

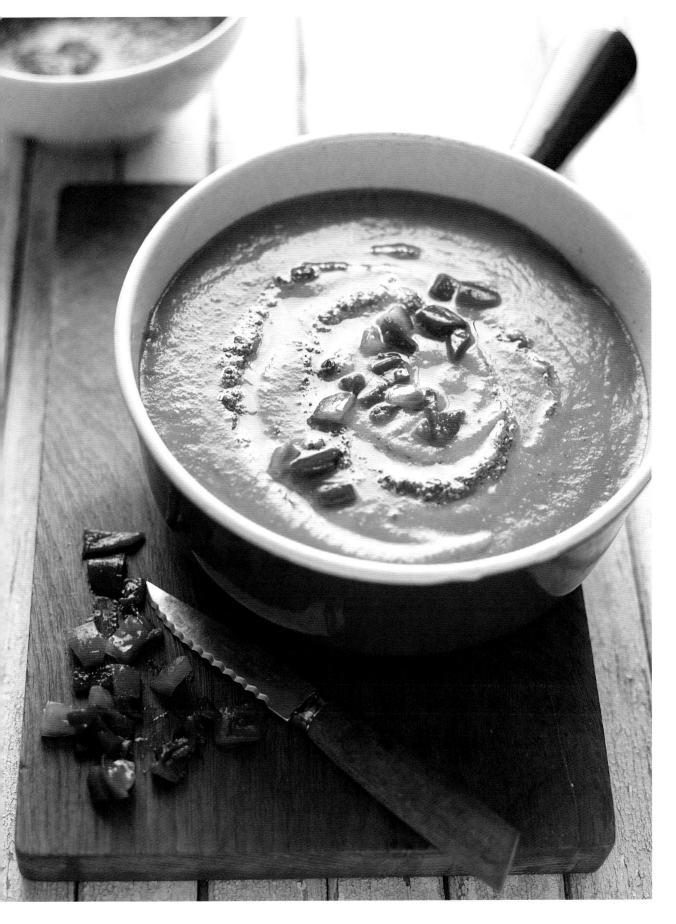

lettuce & dill soup

Serves: 2
Preparation time: 10 minutes
Cooking time: 20 minutes
Wheat free, Gluten free, Vegetarian

Lettuce needn't be confined to the salad bowl. It is also an excellent soup ingredient, especially when paired with dill. This recipe came from Gaby Melvin whose adventurous palate is always proving me wrong!

2 teaspoons olive oil
1 large onion, peeled and thinly sliced
150g potato, peeled and finely diced

Add the oil, onions and potato to medium non-stick pan and stir to coat the vegetables with the oil. Cook over a medium heat and then cover the pan and leave to sweat for 8 minutes.

500ml vegetable stock
Freshly ground black pepper
Pinch grated nutmeg

Add the stock, bring to the boil, season with pepper and nutmeg, and reduce the heat to simmer for 4 minutes.

2 small heads round or 1 iceberg lettuce, finely shredded

Add the lettuce and simmer for 7 more minutes.

2 tablespoons finely chopped fresh dill

Add the dill and allow to cook for a further minute. Blend the soup until smooth, using a hand-held blender or by transferring to a food processor. Strain it through a sieve back into the pan.

3 tablespoons half-fat crème fraîche
Freshly ground black pepper

Add the crème fraîche and stir through gently, then season with black pepper.

To serve
2 teaspoons finely chopped fresh dill
2 slices rye bread (optional)
Half-fat cream cheese (optional)

Ladle the soup into warmed bowls and sprinkle the dill on top. Serve with rye bread spread with a little cream cheese if you like.

TIP Add a touch of luxury by sprinkling over a little diced smoked salmon over the soup. Add a generous grinding of black pepper and a good squeeze of lemon juice to bring the flavours together.

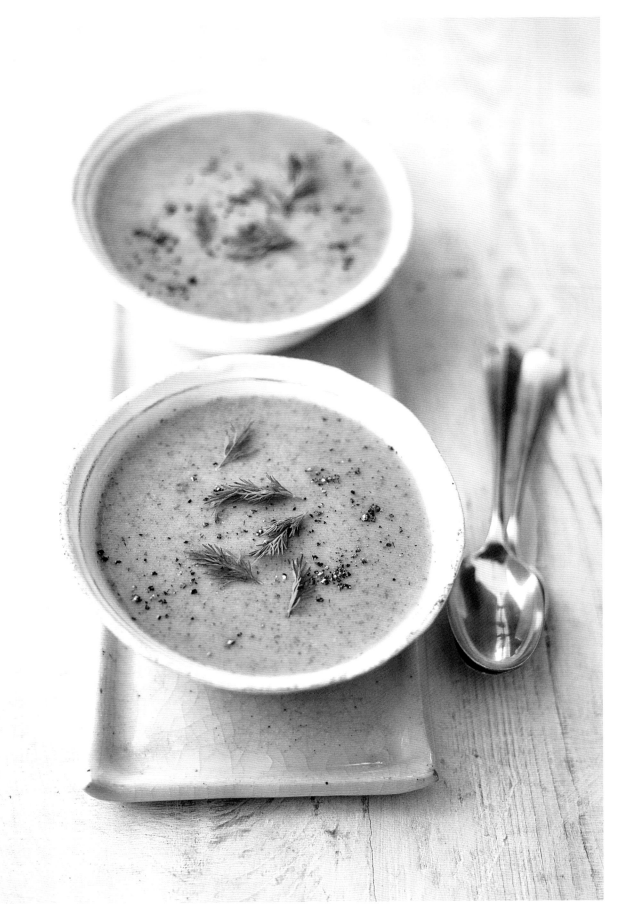

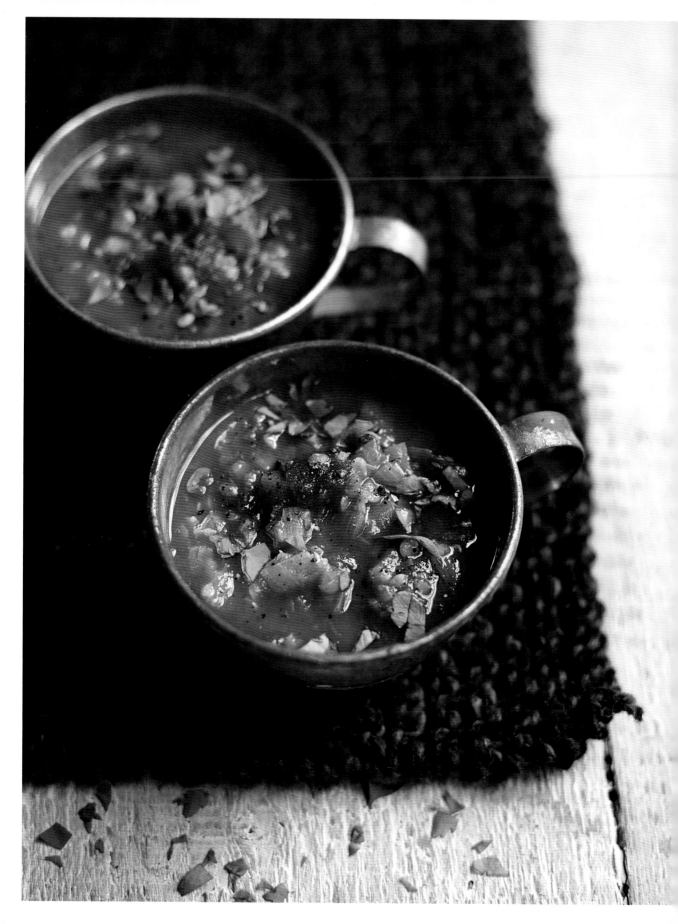

chunky red lentil soup

Serves: 2
Preparation time: 5 minutes
Cooking time: 25 minutes
Wheat free, Gluten free, Dairy free, Vegetarian

A real winner when the cupboards are bare, this warming winter soup is also packed full of vitamins. It involves little more effort than chopping vegetables, mixing the ingredients, and leaving them to their own devices on the stove-top.

2 teaspoons groundnut oil
50g cubed pancetta
1 medium onion, peeled and roughly chopped

1 large carrot, peeled and roughly chopped

75g dried red lentils, rinsed and drained
400g tin chopped tomatoes
400ml vegetable stock

To serve
Freshly ground black pepper
Small handful flat-leaf parsley, finely chopped

Add the oil to a medium-sized non-stick saucepan and place over a medium heat. Add the pancetta and fry for 2 minutes, followed by the onions. Leave to sweat for about 4–5 minutes, stirring occasionally.

Add the carrot and stir to mix with the onion. Cover and leave for another 4–5 minutes, shaking the pan occasionally to prevent sticking.

Add the lentils and tomatoes (along with their juices), then the stock. Bring to the boil, then reduce the heat so the soup simmers steadily.

Cover the pan and leave for 10–15 minutes, or until the lentils have collapsed and the vegetables are soft.

Season the soup with black pepper, then ladle into warmed serving bowls.

Sprinkle with the parsley and serve immediately.

TIP This recipe works well with almost any root vegetable, so get creative. Replace the carrot with sweet potatoes, parsnips or celeriac.

curried parsnip & coconut soup

Serves: 2
Preparation time: 10 minutes
Cooking time: 20 minutes
Wheat free, Gluten free, Dairy free, Vegetarian

This nutty and sweet soup is the perfect way to introduce parsnip to anyone who might be reluctant to try it, and has the added benefits of being a great source of dietary fibre and potassium.

2 teaspoons groundnut oil
1 teaspoon cumin seeds
1 teaspoon caraway seeds

300g parsnips, peeled and cut into small dice
1 small onion, finely chopped
1 celery stalk, finely chopped
2cm piece fresh ginger, peeled and finely chopped
½ teaspoon red chilli flakes
½ teaspoon turmeric
½ teaspoon garam masala
2 tablespoons water

500ml chicken stock
100ml half-fat coconut milk
1 bay leaf
½ teaspoon finely chopped fresh thyme

50g raw cashew nuts

To serve
1 teaspoon finely chopped fresh coriander
Freshly ground black pepper

Heat the oil in a medium non-stick pan and lightly fry the seeds until they start to pop.

Add the parsnips, onion, celery, ginger, chilli flakes, turmeric, garam masala and water. Place the lid on and cook until the onion and celery are soft – about 5 minutes – stirring it every so often to make sure it doesn't stick.

Add the stock, coconut milk, bay leaf and thyme to the pan, then cover and bring to the boil. Reduce the heat and remove the lid, then leave to simmer until all the vegetables are cooked – about 8 minutes.

Stir in the cashew nuts and blend the soup until smooth, using a hand-held blender or by transferring to a food processor.

Ladle into warmed soup bowls and garnish with coriander. Season with black pepper and serve.

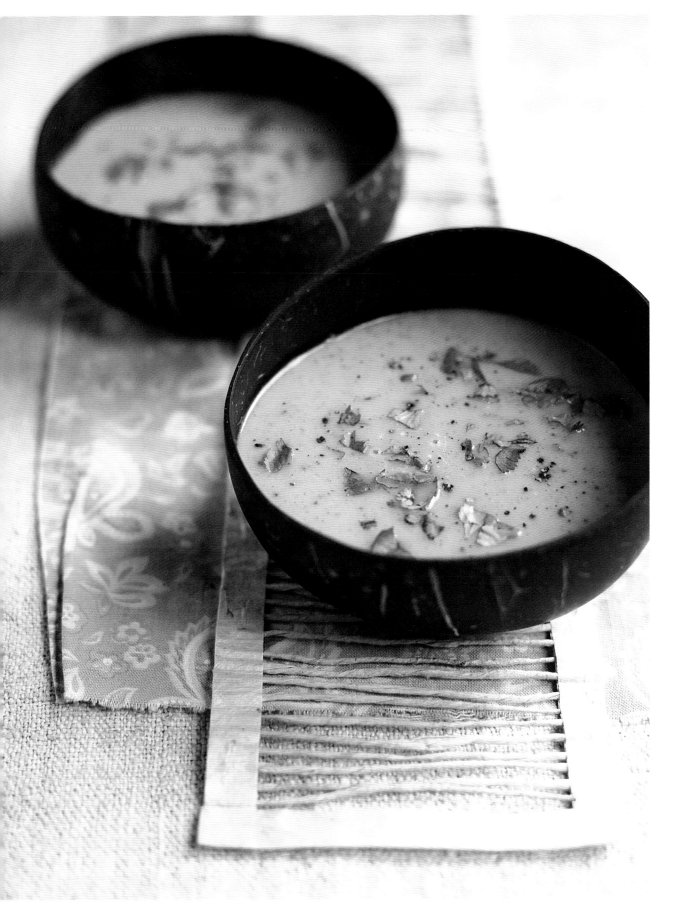

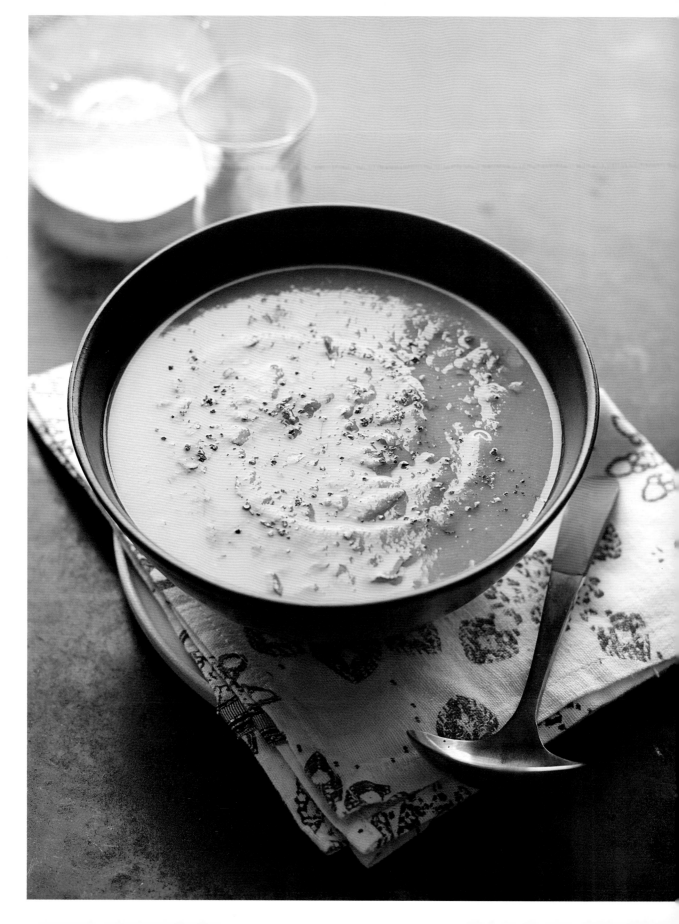

fragrant sweet potato & lime soup

Serves: 2
Preparation time: 10 minutes
Cooking time: 25 minutes
Wheat free, Gluten free, Dairy free, Vegetarian

My friend Jess, a food blogger, made this with carrot, which was utterly fresh and delicious. Although I've used sweet potato and added a few shortcuts, it is still just as gorgeous as the original.

2 teaspoons groundnut oil
1 small onion, peeled and finely chopped

1 garlic clove, peeled and finely chopped
2cm piece fresh ginger, peeled and finely chopped

1 large or 2 small sweet potatoes (about 200g), peeled and diced
500ml chicken or vegetable stock

100g firm tofu, chopped into small dice
2 tablespoons finely chopped fresh coriander

Juice of ½ lime
Freshly ground black pepper

To serve
1 tablespoon finely chopped fresh coriander

Heat the oil in a large non-stick saucepan over a medium heat. Add the onion and leave to sweat for about 3 minutes.

Add the garlic and ginger. Stir to mix the ingredients and leave for a further 1–2 minutes.

Add the sweet potatoes, stir to combine and add the stock. Bring to the boil, then reduce the heat and leave to simmer for about 15 minutes until the potatoes have softened.

Add the tofu and coriander, then blend the soup until smooth, using a hand-held blender or food processor.

Stir in the lime juice, season to taste with black pepper, and warm through before serving.

Ladle the soup into warmed bowls and sprinkle with coriander.

pear & celeriac soup

Serves 2
Preparation time: 15 minutes
Cooking time: 25 minutes
Wheat free, Gluten free, Vegetarian

You might cringe at the thought of fruit in a savoury soup, but the sweetness of the pear perfectly balances the earthiness of the celeriac. This is also a great way to use up pears which might be past their prime.

2 teaspoons groundnut oil
1 small onion, peeled and finely diced

Heat the oil in a large non-stick saucepan over a medium heat and sweat the onions for 3 minutes.

150g celeriac (about half a head), peeled and chopped into small dice
1 celery stalk, finely sliced
30g baby potatoes, chopped into small dice
1 garlic clove, roughly chopped

Add the celeriac, celery, potatoes and garlic. Increase the heat slightly and cook for a further 5 minutes, stirring occasionally.

1 teaspoon curry powder

Add the curry powder and stir well until all of the vegetables are coated.

1 ripe pear, stalk and core removed, finely diced
2 sprigs fresh thyme, leaves picked
1 bay leaf
500ml vegetable stock

Leave the mixture to cook for 2 minutes, before adding the pear, thyme leaves, bay leaf and vegetable stock. Bring to the boil, cover, reduce the heat and simmer for 15 minutes.

2 tablespoons ground almonds

Stir in the almonds. If you have a hand-held blender, blend the soup in the pan. Otherwise, transfer it to a food processor and blend thoroughly.

To serve
20g half-fat crème fraîche

Ladle the soup into bowls and serve with a dollop of crème fraîche on top.

TIP This soup also works well with apples instead of pears. Just replace the pear with a peeled, cored and finely diced apple.

cauliflower cheese soup

Serves: 2
Preparation time: 10 minutes
Cooking time: 20 minutes
Wheat free, Gluten free, Vegetarian

Preparing the classic dish of cauliflower cheese in soup form means that you get all of the velvety, creamy taste but with fewer calories – and a lot less effort.

2 teaspoons groundnut oil
1 medium onion, peeled and roughly chopped
1 garlic clove, peeled and finely sliced

1 medium potato, peeled and diced
½ head of cauliflower, stalks and florets roughly chopped
500ml vegetable stock

30g Parmesan cheese, finely grated
30g mature Cheddar cheese, finely grated

To serve
Freshly ground black pepper
2 tablespoons half-fat crème fraîche
Small handful flat-leaf parsley, finely chopped

Add the oil, onion and garlic to a medium saucepan, over a medium heat. Cover and leave to soften for 5 minutes, stirring occasionally.

Stir in the potato and cauliflower. Add the vegetable stock and bring to the boil. Cover and reduce the heat so that the soup simmers steadily for 15 minutes.

Transfer the soup to a food processor (or use a hand-held blender) and blend until smooth.

Return to the saucepan, heat through, then add the Parmesan and Cheddar in a steady flow, stirring constantly so that it melts through the soup completely.

Season the soup with pepper, then ladle into warmed serving bowls. Dollop a spoonful of crème fraîche into each bowl and sprinkle with the parsley.

gazpacho

Serves: 2
Preparation time: 10 minutes
Wheat free, Gluten free, Vegetarian
Place serving bowls in the fridge to cool

This zingy, cool Spanish soup will perk you up on a hot day. Simply blend the raw ingredients and you're left with a delicious soup that's packed with antioxidants and vitamins A and C.

1 spring onion, trimmed and roughly chopped
4 tomatoes, roughly chopped
½ red pepper, deseeded and roughly chopped
⅓ cucumber, peeled and roughly chopped
1 small garlic clove, peeled and crushed
Small handful fresh basil leaves

Put the spring onion, tomatoes, red pepper, cucumber, garlic and basil in a blender, and blitz until completely smooth – about 2 minutes of continuous blending.

Juice of ½ lemon
1 tablespoon extra virgin olive oil
Freshly ground black pepper

Add the lemon juice, olive oil and pepper, and stir to mix. Taste and adjust seasoning where necessary. If the soup seems too thick, add a couple of tablespoons of water and stir through.

To serve
4 ice cubes
Few basil leaves, roughly chopped
50g feta cheese, crumbled (optional)

Place 2 ice cubes into each chilled bowl, divide the soup between the bowls, and sprinkle with basil leaves and feta (if using).

TIP For a sharper taste, replace the lemon juice with 2 tablespoons of red wine vinegar.

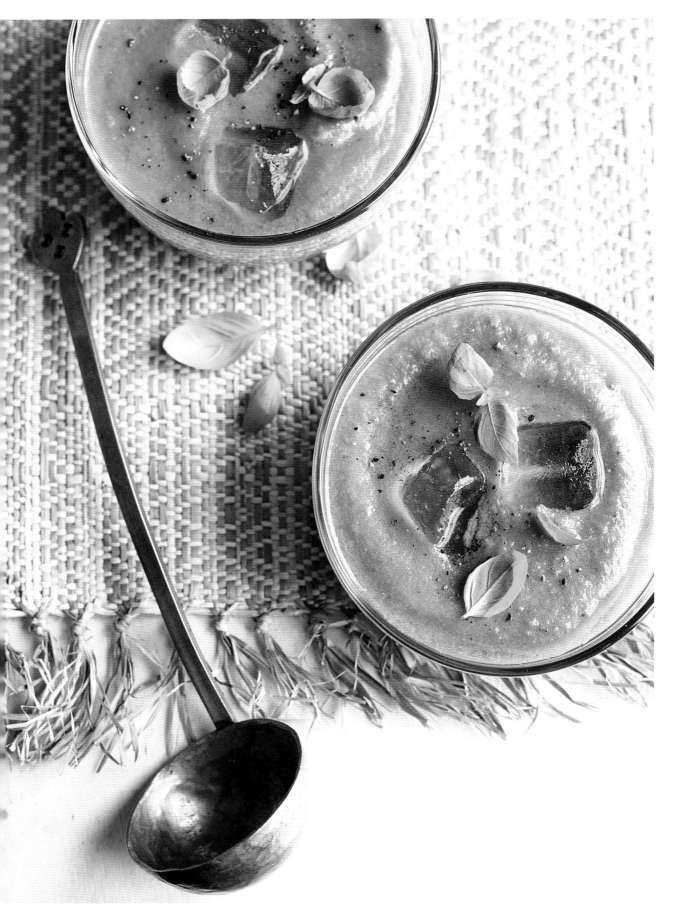

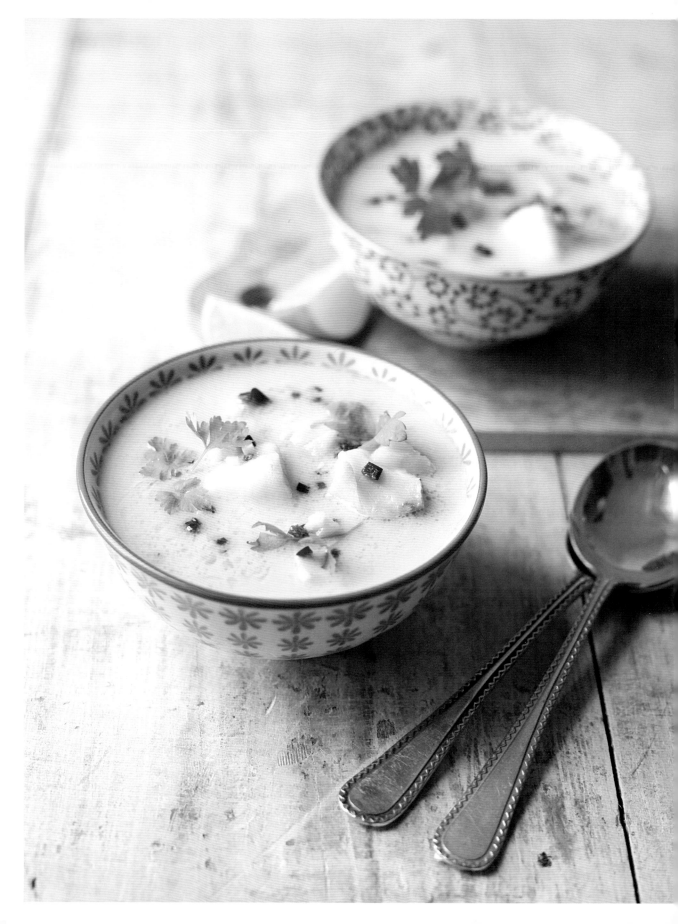

coconut fish soup

Serves: 2
Preparation time: 10 minutes
Cooking time: 15 minutes
Wheat free, Gluten free, Dairy free

Super-quick to make, this soup is little more than fish poached in a zesty coconut broth. The aromatic herbs and spices add a wonderful depth of flavour.

400ml vegetable stock
200ml half-fat coconut milk
½ jalapeño chilli, diced
1cm piece fresh ginger, peeled and finely chopped

Place the stock, coconut milk, chilli and ginger in a medium non-stick pan and bring to the boil.

80g thick rice noodles

Put the noodles in a bowl of just-boiled water and leave to soak for 10 minutes or according to the packet instructions. When the noodles are soft, but still have bite, drain well and set aside.

160g mixed filleted white fish (such as hake, cod, haddock or pollock), skinned and cut into small chunks

Reduce the heat to a simmer, and add the fish. Cook for about 3 minutes, until the fish is cooked through.

Juice of ½ lime

Add the lime juice and leave to simmer for a further 2 minutes.

To serve
Small handful fresh coriander leaves

Divide the noodles between 2 deep serving bowls. Ladle over the soup, and sprinkle with the coriander.

aromatic chicken & corn noodle soup

A comfort-food classic – chicken and noodle soup – is given a South East Asian twist here. The ginger, lime and fish sauce are a perfect match for the bland warmth of a wholesome noodle soup. Definitely one to curl up with on the sofa.

Serves: 2
Preparation time: 10 minutes
Cooking time: 25 minutes
Wheat free, Gluten free, Dairy free

1 tablespoon groundnut oil
2 spring onions, trimmed and chopped (retain the green bits)
½ red chilli, deseeded and finely chopped
2cm piece fresh ginger, peeled and finely sliced
1 garlic clove, peeled and finely sliced

Add the oil, spring onions, chilli, ginger and garlic to a medium non-stick pan and place over a low heat. Stir until soft – about 2 minutes.

500ml chicken or vegetable stock

Add the stock and bring to the boil.

1 small chicken breast, skin removed

Add the chicken breast. Reduce the heat, cover and simmer for 12–15 minutes, or until the chicken is cooked through. Remove the chicken to a plate and shred it finely, then return to the pan.

50g vermicelli rice noodles
195g tin sweetcorn kernels, drained
½ teaspoon Thai fish sauce
2 teaspoons tamari soy sauce

Add the noodles, sweetcorn, fish sauce, soy sauce and the retained green leaves of the spring onions, and simmer for about 3 minutes until the noodles are soft (or follow the instructions on the noodle packet).

Juice of ½ lime
Small handful fresh coriander, roughly chopped

Stir through the lime juice and coriander.

To serve
2 lime wedges (optional)
Small handful fresh coriander leaves

Divide the noodles between 2 serving bowls, then ladle the soup, chicken and vegetables over the top. Garnish with the lime wedges (if using) and additional coriander. Serve immediately.

TIP To make a vegetarian version, omit the fish sauce and chicken and replace with an extra dash of tamari soy sauce and 100g firm tofu, cut into cubes – add this with the noodles and vegetables.

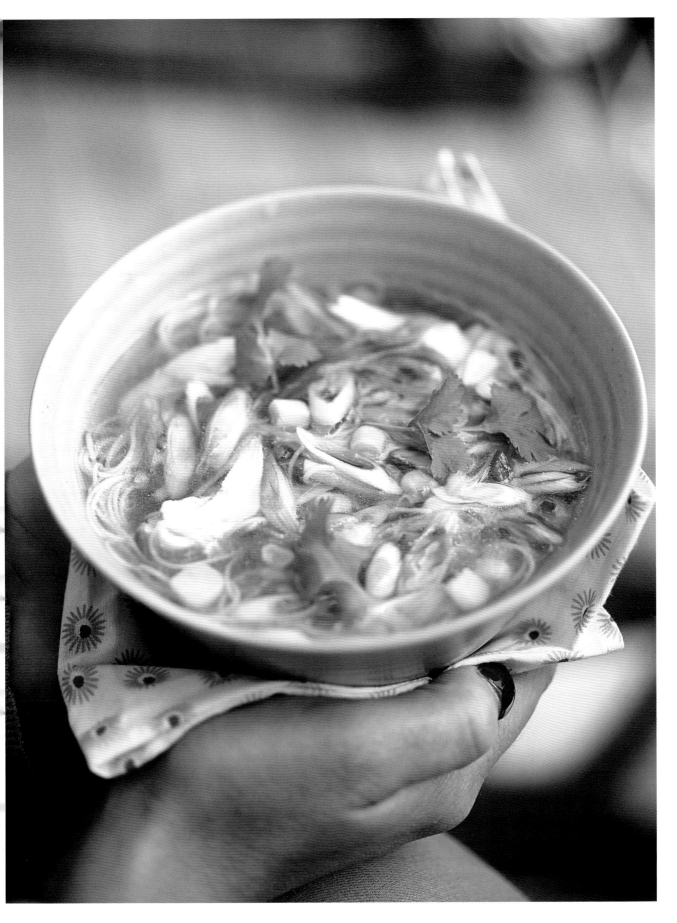

mains

pesto 98

caramelised red onion & goat's cheese frittata 100

courgette, butter bean & feta cakes 102

new potato & cream cheese frittata 104

red mullet 'en papillote' 106

soy-glazed salmon 108

speedy fish pie 110

king prawn thai yellow curry 112

chicken & asparagus with coriander pesto 114

mushrooms stuffed with
courgettes & goat's cheese 116

chicken in whole spices 117

turmeric chicken skewers 118

jerk chicken 120

steak with peppercorn sauce 121

grilled lamb cutlets with mint raita 122

blue cheese burgers 124

beef & broccoli in oyster sauce 126

SPEEDY and fuss-free mains that are delicious enough for the whole family have transformed my busy days. While it needs to be quick and easy to prepare, the main should also be packed with energy-giving goodness. The recipes that follow are full of whole foods, grains and quality proteins that will really help take care of you and your family.

In each main, you will find that the protein element – fish, meat or pulse – takes centre-stage. This ensures that, with one of the carb sides and a couple of vegetable sides, you have a fully balanced, well-rounded plate of food.

Adding fresh herbs and spices also plays an essential part in enhancing other ingredients, not to mention being a great additional source of nutrients. A variation in spices can take a humble piece of chicken wherever you want to go: from Mexico to Texas or across the globe to India or Thailand.

The convenience and flexible nature of these recipes will help you create something marvellous with minimal effort. And thanks to upcycling, most of these meals can also transform busy lunchtimes the following day.

pesto

Serves: 4–6
Preparation time: 10 minutes
Wheat free, Gluten free, Vegetarian

Pesto is a lifesaver for the time-poor cook. It can quickly transform basic ingredients into an instant dish, which is why I have included it in the mains chapter. What's more, the herbs in pesto are stuffed full of nutrients. Both basil and coriander are excellent sources of vitamins A and K, while mint is full of vitamin C. Oil and garlic are added to the herbs, as well as calcium-dense cheeses and nuts packed with vitamin E, making pesto a real superfood. Classic pesto is made with basil, pine nuts, garlic, Parmesan and olive oil, but the basic notion of pesto – a nutty seed pulverised with herbs, hard cheese and oil – is ideal for experimenting with.

Although you can follow tradition and use a pestle and mortar, I find that using a food processor or blender is far quicker. However, increase the quantities by half to achieve a smoother and more even texture. Any excess pesto will refrigerate or freeze well (see Storage Tips below).

STORAGE TIPS

Pesto will keep well in your fridge for 4 days; for longer-term storage, spoon the pesto into an ice-cube tray and freeze. I like to pop the frozen cubes out of the tray and keep them in ziplock bags in the freezer. A cube will defrost quickly: in the time it takes to boil water for pasta, the cube is almost room temperature again.

basil pesto

100g basil leaves
40g pine nuts
80g Parmesan cheese, freshly grated
1 tablespoon olive oil
1 garlic clove

Place all the ingredients in a food processor or blender and blitz until you have a stiff paste.

mint pesto

40g walnuts
3 garlic cloves, peeled
60g mint leaves
100g feta cheese
1 tablespoon lemon juice

Place all the ingredients in a food processor or blender and blitz until you have a stiff paste.

coriander pesto

1 tablespoon coriander seeds

40g unsalted cashew nuts
60g fresh coriander
1 green chilli, deseeded and chopped
2 tablespoons olive oil
2 tablespoons finely grated
Parmesan cheese

Toast the coriander seeds in a dry, non-stick frying pan, shaking occasionally, until they are browned but not burnt.

Mix the remaining ingredients in a blender until you have a smooth paste.

SERVING SUGGESTIONS

- Stir a portion of coriander pesto through cooked rice noodles and serve alongside a piece of grilled fish.

- Pan-fry a handful of prawns and some finely sliced asparagus in a non-stick pan with a dash of groundnut oil, add a tablespoon of pesto of your choice per serving and heat through.

- Spread pesto on top of toasted rye bread and top with grilled asparagus or avocado slices.

- Dollop a few teaspoons of basil or mint pesto onto an omelette while cooking and top with cheese.

- Add a spoonful of mint or basil pesto to warm new potatoes and stir through. Serve hot or cold.

- Use olive oil to thin the pesto down and use as a dressing for any simple salad.

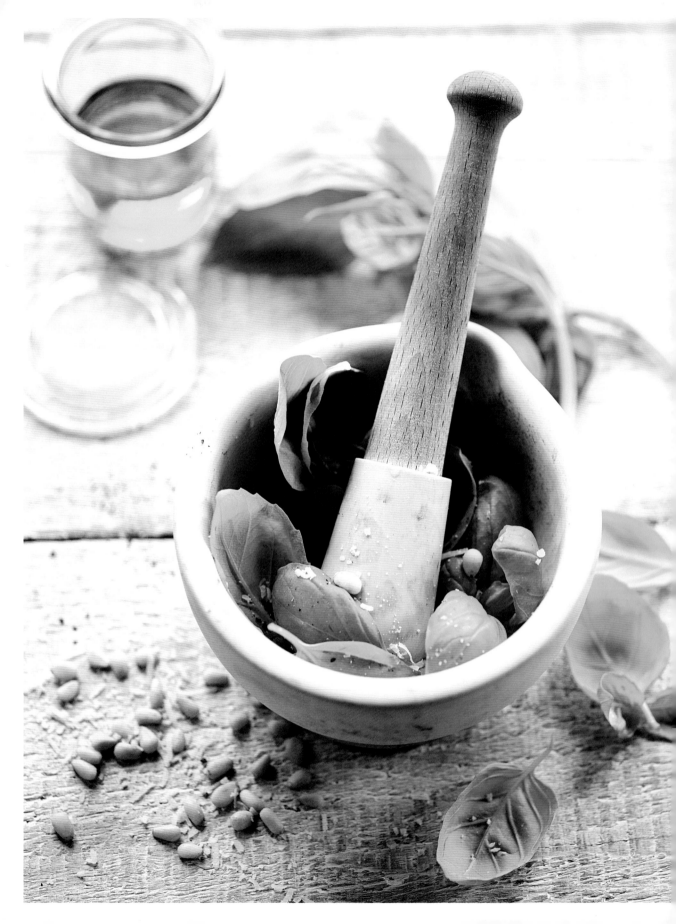

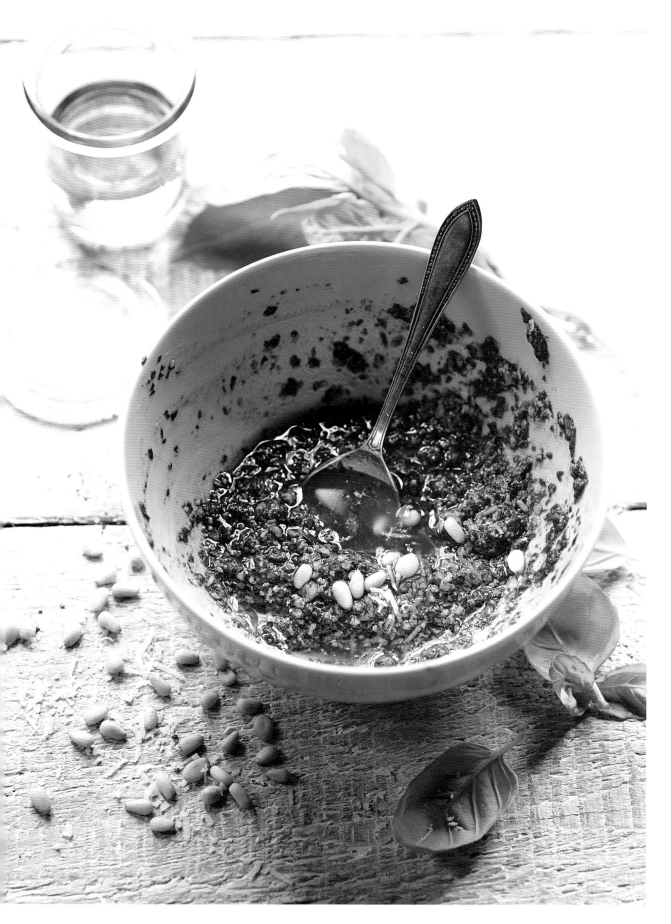

caramelised red onion and goat's cheese frittata

Serves: 2
Preparation time: 5 minutes
Cooking time: 20 minutes
Wheat free, Gluten free, Vegetarian
Preheat grill to high

Frittatas are a good throw-together meal. Substitute the goat's cheese for feta or Cheddar if you like.

2 teaspoons groundnut oil
1 red onion, peeled and finely sliced

Add the oil to the pan with the onion and sweat on a low–medium heat with the lid on for about 10 minutes, or until they begin to soften and brown a little at the edges.

3 large free-range eggs
Freshly ground black pepper

Meanwhile, crack the eggs into a bowl and beat with a fork, then add some black pepper.

Pour the eggs into the pan and cook for a further 5–6 minutes, until the eggs are almost set.

100g goat's cheese

Break the goat's cheese into rough chunks and dot over the top.

Place the frittata under the hot grill for 3 minutes, then shake to check that the egg is set firm while the cheese is soft and bubbling. Pop it back under the grill for another minute or so if needed.

To serve
Large handful rocket leaves
1 ready-cooked beetroot, diced
Balsamic vinegar

Serve topped with rocket, beetroot and a drizzle of balsamic vinegar.

UPCYCLE The frittata can be enjoyed cold the next day accompanied by sliced red pepper and cucumber.

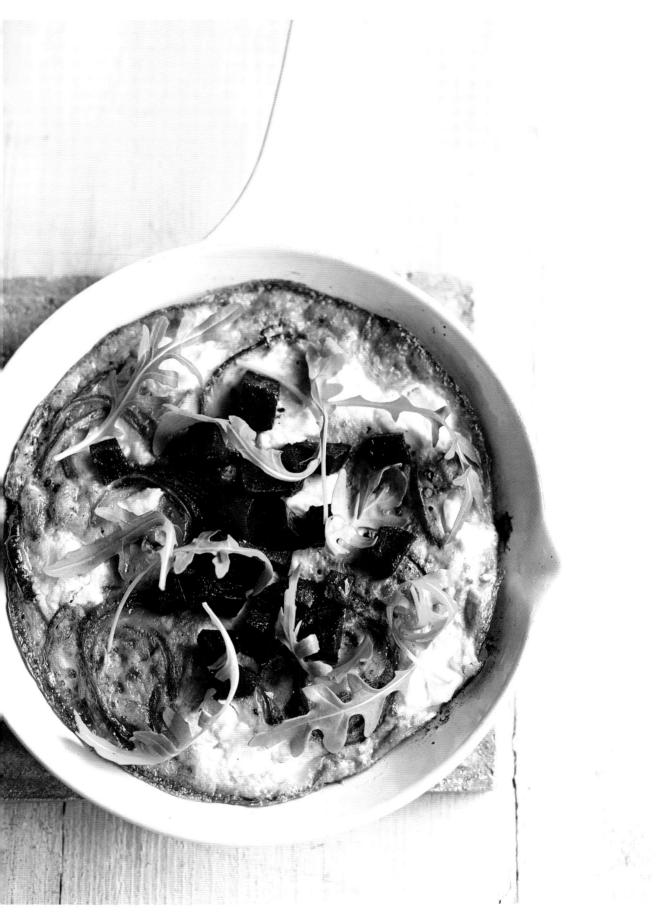

courgette, butter bean & feta cakes

These scrumptious little cakes can be enjoyed a multitude of ways. As well as being the focal point of a lovely dinner, they also make a delectable sandwich filling (see Upcycle).

Serves: 2
Preparation time: 15 minutes (including chilling time)
Cooking time: 20 minutes
Wheat free, Gluten free, Vegetarian
Preheat oven to 220°C/425°F/Gas mark 7, and place a non-stick baking tray inside

1 large courgette

Coarsely grate the courgette, then scoop up the pieces in your hands and firmly squeeze all of the liquid from them. (It's important that the courgette is as dry as possible so that the cakes aren't soggy or bitter.) Leave to drain in a colander and squeeze dry again if necessary.

120g tin butter beans, drained and rinsed
50g feta cheese, crumbled
1 handful fresh basil, finely chopped
1 spring onion, trimmed and finely chopped

In a large bowl, roughly mash the butter beans, then add the courgette, feta, basil and spring onion. Mix together well.

Using your hands, divide the mixture and form into small patties, and place in the fridge for 10 minutes to chill.

2 teaspoons groundnut oil

Coat a non-stick frying pan with oil and remove any excess oil with kitchen paper. Fry the patties over a medium heat for about 1 minute on each side.

Transfer the patties to the hot tray in the oven and bake for 10 minutes.

225g tin chopped tomatoes
2 tablespoons half-fat crème fraîche
½ teaspoon tamari soy sauce
½ teaspoon balsamic vinegar

Meanwhile, add the tomatoes to a small saucepan and warm on a medium heat to break them up. Once the tomatoes are warmed through, take off the heat and stir through the crème fraîche, soy sauce and vinegar. Then blend until smooth using a hand-held blender or transfer to a food processor.

To serve
Basil leaves

Remove the patties from the oven and serve with the tomato sauce on the side and a garnish of basil leaves.

⬈ UPCYCLE Any leftover courgette cakes can be stuffed into pitta bread, spread with hummus and filled with salad leaves, chopped tomatoes and cucumber. Add a dollop of crème fraîche if you like.

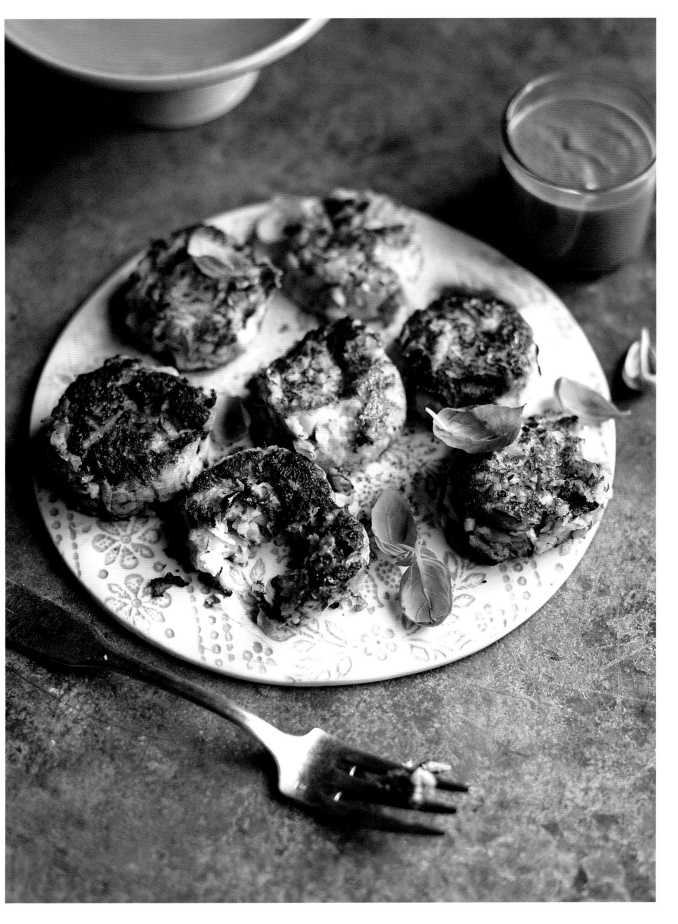

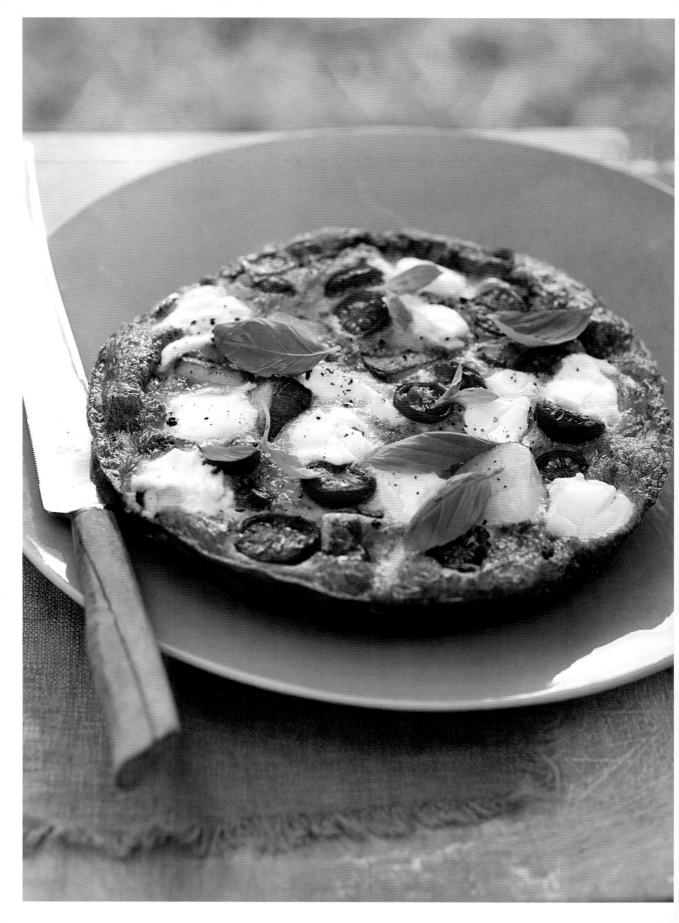

new potato & cream cheese frittata

Because this dish relies on speedy cooking and assembly, try to have everything lined up and ready to hand before you start.

Serves: 2
Preparation time: 10 minutes
Cooking time: 15 minutes
Wheat free, Gluten free, Vegetarian
Preheat grill to high

200g new potatoes, cut into quarters	Add the new potatoes to a pan of boiling water and cook until softened.
4 large free-range eggs Freshly ground black pepper	Meanwhile, crack the eggs into a bowl and beat with a fork, then add some black pepper to the mixture.
	Drain the potatoes and slice into 1cm thick pieces.
1 teaspoon groundnut oil	Heat the oil in an ovenproof non-stick pan and add the drained potatoes. Cook until they are brown.
10 cherry tomatoes, halved	Pour the egg mixture into the pan and then add the tomatoes, cut side up.
100g half-fat cream cheese	Dollop the cream cheese over the top of the frittata.
	Cook in the pan until the mixture starts to set and the egg starts to brown underneath.
	Pop the frittata under the hot grill for about 3 minutes.
	Remove from the grill and shake the pan. The eggs should be firmly set, and the cream cheese soft and runny. Pop it back under the grill for another minute or so, if needed. When ready to serve, flip the frittata out on to the plate.
To serve Basil leaves	Garnish with basil leaves before serving, then cut into wedges.

⚡ UPCYCLE This makes the perfect next-day food. If you want to make it in advance to have the following day, try using a hard cheese such as Parmesan or pecorino. Simply serve it with a handful of sugar snaps and some cherry tomatoes for a satisfying lunch.

105

red mullet 'en papillote'

Serves: 2
Preparation time: 10 minutes
Cooking time: 15 minutes
Wheat free, Gluten free, Dairy free
Preheat oven to 220°C/425°F/Gas mark 7, and place a non-stick baking tray inside

Cooking fish 'en papillote' is simpler than it sounds. Ingredients are popped into a paper or foil parcel and baked. Just remember to seal the parcels well so that you retain the wonderful juices.

1 teaspoon olive oil
2 red mullet fillets, deboned, cleaned and trimmed

Freshly ground black pepper
4 sprigs thyme

Brush two large squares of foil or baking parchment with a little olive oil, then place the fish diagonally across the centre of it.

Season the fish and place a couple sprigs of thyme on top of each fillet.

Now bring the edges of the paper together and fold over to form a parcel, leaving a section open.

25ml white wine
4 tablespoons lemon juice
2 sprigs fresh thyme
Freshly ground black pepper
1 lemon, cut into slices

In a small bowl, mix together the wine, lemon juice, thyme and black pepper. Spoon the dressing into each parcel, dividing it equally between them. Tuck a few lemon slices into each parcel too.

Seal the parcels well by folding the foil or paper over on itself two or three times, then place on the heated baking tray and bake for 10–12 minutes. (After 10 minutes, check the fish for doneness – it should be opaque.)

To serve

Put the unopened parcels straight on to warmed plates and serve at the table, allowing each person to open their own.

TIP Almost any type of firm fish can be cooked in this way; the cooking time will vary according to the thickness of the fish. Try it with salmon, trout, sea bass or even prawns.

UPCYCLE Red mullet makes a tasty topping for couscous or quinoa. Simply prepare your grain, add some diced tomatoes, cucumber and herbs of your choice, and top with the fish for an easy and satisfying salad.

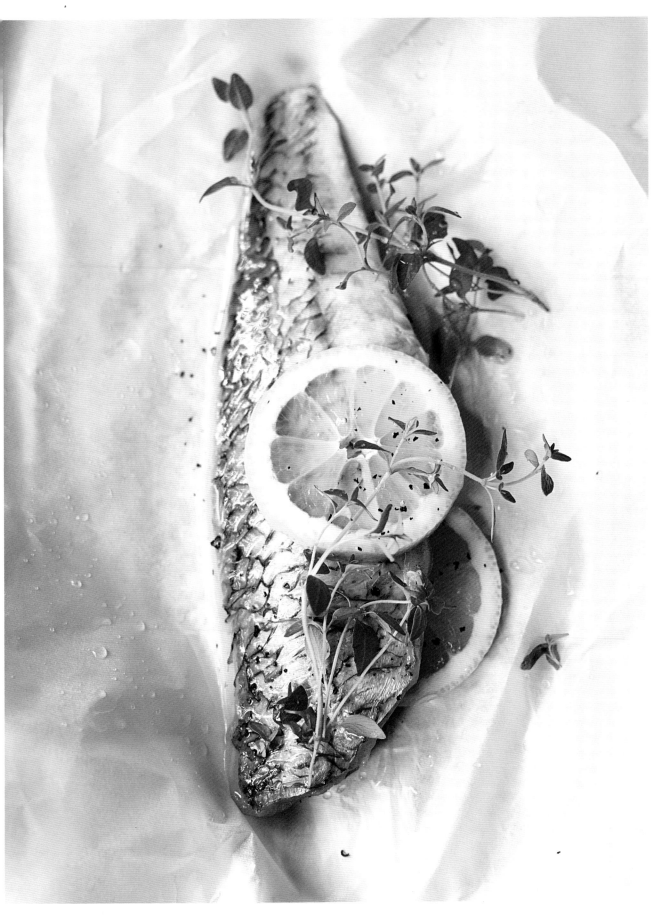

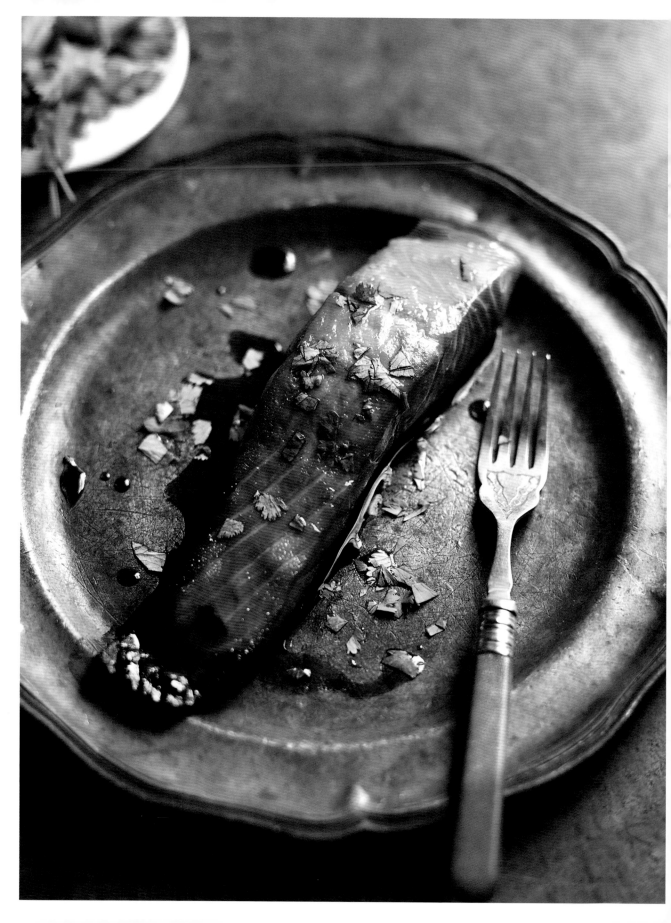

soy-glazed salmon

This is a fantastically delicious and simple dish, which will appeal to even the most picky of eaters. If my children ever complain about eating fish, this recipe always wins them back!

Serves: 2
Preparation time: 5 minutes
Cooking time: 20 minutes
Wheat free, Gluten free, Dairy free
Preheat oven to 180°C/350°F/Gas mark 4, and place an ovenproof dish inside

2 tablespoons tamari soy sauce
2 tablespoons honey
2 tablespoons lemon or lime juice

2 x 100g salmon fillets, skinned

Make the marinade by mixing together the soy sauce, honey and lemon or lime juice.

Place the salmon fillets in a small bowl and spoon over the marinade, turning the fish so that it is nicely covered. Leave to sit for 10 minutes, before transferring to the hot ovenproof dish.

Place in the oven for around 15 minutes or until the fish is cooked through.

To serve
2 teaspoons finely chopped fresh coriander

Remove from the oven and serve on individual plates, pouring over the sauce and garnishing with coriander. Eat immediately.

TIP If you like a bit of heat, add half a red chilli, deseeded and finely chopped, to the marinade.

UPCYCLE Cook more salmon than you need to create the basis of some wonderful lunch recipes. Simply place the cold salmon on top of a bed of baby spinach with finely sliced carrots, cucumber and sugar snaps, along with segments of grapefruit. Serve with a drizzle of soy sauce.

109

speedy fish pie

A shortcut on the traditional fish pie, which can take an hour or more to cook in the oven, this recipe simply requires cooking the individual components, then popping the dish under the grill for a few minutes.

Serves: 2
Preparation time: 15 minutes
Cooking time: 25 minutes
Wheat free, Gluten free
Preheat grill to high

200g small baby potatoes, unpeeled and halved

Cook the potatoes in a pan of boiling water for 10–15 minutes until tender.

1 teaspoon groundnut oil
½ onion, peeled and finely diced (retain the trimmings)
1 leek, washed and finely sliced (white part only; retain the trimmings and the dark green leaves)
1 garlic clove, peeled and crushed
½ celery stalk, chopped into small dice
1 carrot, peeled and chopped into small dice

While the potatoes are cooking, place the groundnut oil, onion, leek, garlic, celery and carrot in a non-stick pan. Sweat over a medium heat for 10 minutes, lid on, stirring occasionally to prevent sticking.

100g salmon fillet, skin on, boned
100g white fish fillet (I like pollock or sea bream), skin on, boned
1 bay leaf

Meanwhile, place the fish fillets in a pan with the bay leaf and the leek and onion trimmings, and just cover the mix with hot water. Bring to the boil and then lower the heat. Cover and leave to simmer for about 5 minutes.

Strain the fish, removing the bay leaf and vegetables, and retain the poaching water.

Remove the skin and flake the fish into chunks.

Zest and juice of ½ lemon
100g half-fat crème fraîche
30g Parmesan cheese, grated
Small handful fresh parsley, finely chopped
50g frozen peas
Freshly ground black pepper

Add 2 tablespoons of the poaching water, lemon zest and juice, crème fraîche, Parmesan and half of the parsley to the onion and carrot mix. Add the peas and stir well. Leave for a couple of minutes to heat through, so that the peas defrost, then season with black pepper.

Mix through the flaked fish.

1 teaspoon olive oil

Drain and roughly crush the cooked potatoes with the remainder of the parsley and olive oil. Don't overwork it, as you want the mash to have a nice chunky texture.

15g Parmesan cheese, grated

Spoon the fish and vegetable mix into a deep serving dish. Top with the smashed potatoes and then scatter the Parmesan evenly over the top.

Grill for 5 minutes or until the top is nice and crispy.

TIP Feel free to vary the fish or combination of fish. For special occasions, add a handful of cooked prawns and a little smoked salmon for that extra touch of luxury.

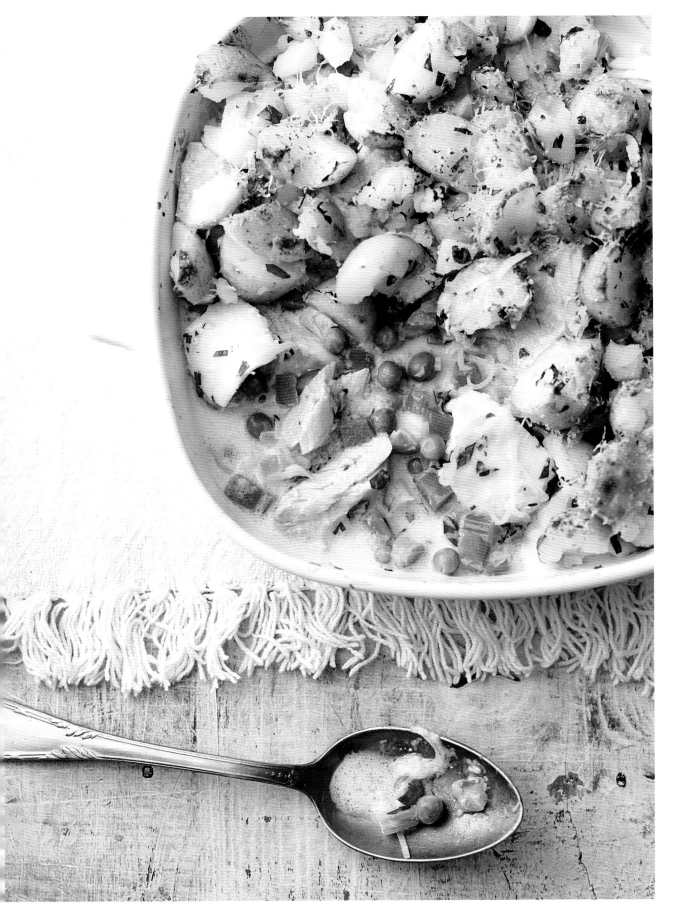

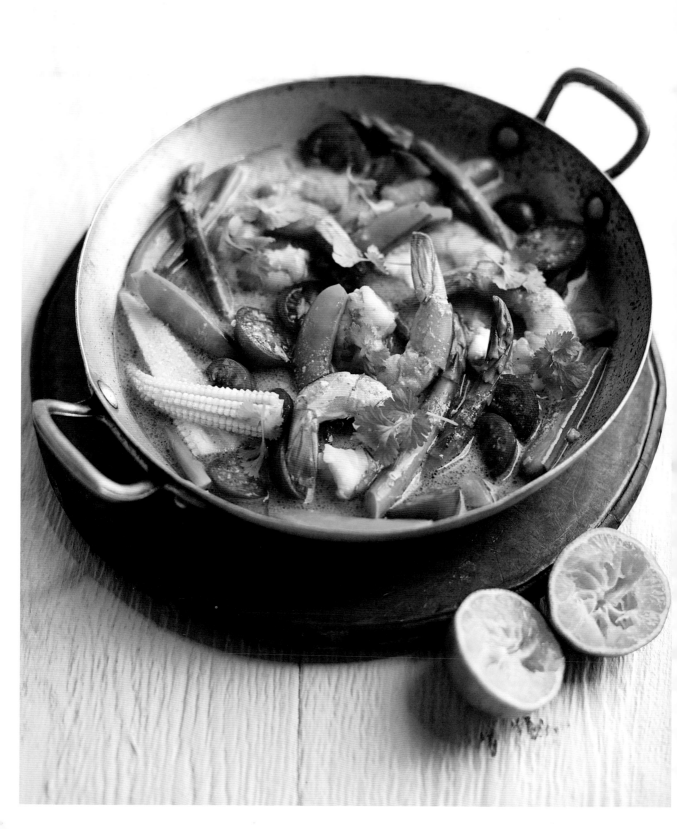

king prawn thai yellow curry

While I usually try to make curries from scratch, sometimes there just isn't time. Good quality ready-made pastes are a fabulous alternative and I promise you won't even notice the difference!

Serves: 2
Preparation time: 10 minutes
Cooking time: 15 minutes
Wheat free, Gluten free, Dairy free

1 teaspoon groundnut oil
2 teaspoons gluten-free Thai yellow
curry paste
1 garlic clove, peeled and finely chopped
1cm piece fresh ginger, peeled
and finely chopped

1 teaspoon Thai fish sauce
2 tablespoons lime juice
250ml half-fat coconut milk
1 tablespoon finely chopped coriander

100g asparagus, fine tips
100g baby corn, halved lengthways
200g sugar snap peas

180g cherry tomatoes, halved
160g raw jumbo king prawns
1 teaspoon lime juice

To serve
2 teaspoons finely chopped coriander

Heat the oil and curry paste in a heavy-based pan over a medium heat. Fry for 1 minute, being careful not to burn the paste. Reduce the heat, add the garlic and ginger and cook for 2 minutes.

Add the fish sauce, lime juice, coconut milk and coriander, and bring to just below boiling.

Tip in the asparagus, baby corn and sugar snap peas, bring to the boil, then reduce the heat and simmer for 4–5 minutes.

Add the tomatoes, followed by the prawns, and cook until the prawns are pink through – this should take about 3 minutes. Add the lime juice and stir through.

Garnish with coriander and eat immediately.

TIP You can replace the prawns with almost any other seafood available, and chicken would also work well. If using fish, choose firm-fleshed fish (such as pollack or kingfish) and cut it into bite-sized pieces.

UPCYCLE To make a delicious soup, simply add 150ml vegetable stock per serving to the curry and stir gently through.

113

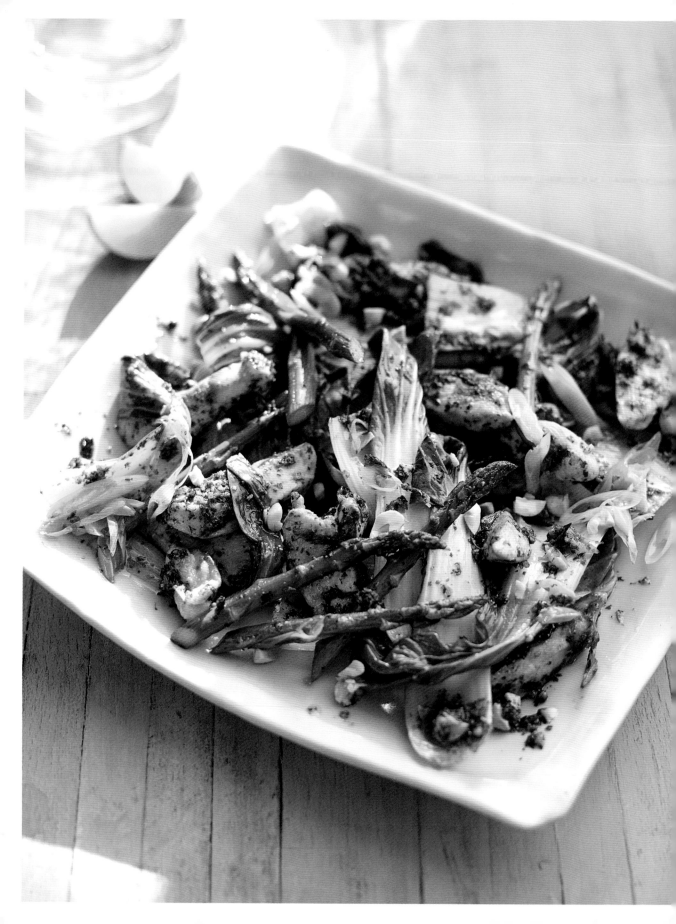

chicken & asparagus with coriander pesto

Serves: 2
Preparation time: 10 minutes
Cooking time: 10 minutes
Wheat free, Gluten free, Dairy free

The coriander pesto in this recipe really brings all the flavours in this stir-fry together. You can also use fish and for a vegetarian version, just substitute the chicken with tofu and steamed vegetables.

2 teaspoons groundnut oil
2 spring onions, trimmed and roughly chopped
200g free-range chicken breasts, skinned and cut into thin strips

100g pak choi or spinach
100g asparagus spears, trimmed

Juice of ½ lime

1 portion Coriander Pesto (page 97)

To serve
Lime wedges
1 tablespoon unsalted cashew nuts, roughly chopped

Heat the oil in a wok or large non-stick pan, then add the spring onions. Stir-fry over a high heat for 3 minutes. Add the chicken strips to the wok.

Once the chicken begins to brown, add the pak choi or spinach and the asparagus.

When the green leaves have started to wilt, add the lime juice. Stir through and take off the heat.

Add the pesto to the chicken mix and place back on the heat for a couple of minutes to warm through. Stir well for a couple of minutes.

Spoon the stir-fry into serving bowls and sprinkle the cashew nuts on top. Serve immediately with lime wedges on the side.

TIP A good rule of thumb for making well-balanced stir-fries is to use two main vegetables and one protein. If asparagus and greens aren't your favourite, mix and match any of the following: broccoli florets, sugar snap peas, thinly sliced carrots, peppers, mushrooms, or even courgette shavings.

⤴ UPCYCLE This recipe makes an excellent open sandwich. Just spread some rye bread with a little of the pesto, then add sliced tomato, a handful of baby leaves and, most importantly, the chopped chicken.

mushrooms stuffed with courgettes & goat's cheese

Goat's cheese and lemongrass are a surprisingly good match. Large field mushrooms are ideal, but you could also use regular mushrooms and serve them as canapes.

Serves: 2
Preparation time: 10 minutes
Cooking time: 25 minutes
Wheat free, Gluten free, Vegetarian
Preheat grill to high

For the lemongrass pesto
1 stalk lemongrass, finely chopped
Zest and juice of 1 lemon
Small handful non-salted macadamia nuts
1 garlic clove, peeled and chopped
3cm piece fresh ginger, peeled and chopped
1 teaspoon coconut flakes
1 tablespoon chopped coriander
1 tablespoon chopped lemon (or regular) basil
1 teaspoon sesame oil
½ red chilli, deseeded and finely chopped

Place all the pesto ingredients in a blender and mix until you have a fine but juicy paste. If it seems too dry, add a teaspoon or two of water until you have a mushy consistency.

4 portobello mushrooms

Rinse the mushrooms and remove and discard the stalks. Place the mushrooms on a non-stick baking tray, cover with tin foil and roast in a hot oven for 15 minutes.

2 teaspoons groundnut oil
1 small onion, peeled and finely chopped
1 garlic clove, peeled and finely chopped

Meanwhile, heat the oil, onion and garlic in a small non-stick pan over a medium heat. Sweat for about 3 minutes, until soft.

120g courgettes, grated and squeezed to drain off all liquid

Add the courgettes, and cook for 10 minutes, until very soft.

Mix in half of the lemongrass pesto, and stir well. (Put the remaining pesto aside for serving.)

80g goat's cheese log, cut into 4 slices

Divide the courgette mix between the roasted mushrooms, then top each one with a slice of goat's cheese. Place under the hot grill for 5–10 minutes, until the cheese is golden and bubbling.

To serve

Place 2 of the mushrooms on each serving plate, and drizzle the remainder of the pesto over the top. Serve immediately.

⊿ UPCYCLE For an almost instant lunch the next day, slice leftovers and serve on top of some cooked noodles that have been tossed through with more of the lemongrass pesto or with sesame oil.

chicken in whole spices

Serves: 2
Preparation time: 10 minutes
Cooking time: 30 minutes
Wheat free, Gluten free, Dairy free
Preheat oven to 200°C/400°F/Gas mark 6

Don't be put off by the long list of spices for this recipe – it's just a matter of lining them up and adding a pinch here and a dash there. This dish goes particularly well with Lemony Creamed Spinach (page 179).

2 cardamom pods
½ cinnamon stick, broken into pieces
1 clove
Pinch ground mace
Pinch cayenne pepper
¼ teaspoon freshly ground black pepper
½ bay leaf, crumbled
½ teaspoon yellow mustard seeds

Shell the cardamom pods, remove the seeds, and grind them together with the cinnamon, clove, mace, cayenne pepper, black pepper, bay leaf and mustard seeds in a pestle and mortar or spice grinder.

1 tablespoon groundnut oil
1 teaspoon turmeric
¼ teaspoon ground ginger

Heat the oil in a large ovenproof pan, add the turmeric and ginger and fry, over a high heat, for 30 seconds.

2 free-range chicken breasts, skinned

Add the chicken, and quickly brown on each side.

1 garlic clove, finely chopped
3 small onions, finely chopped

Add the garlic, onions and the spice mix to the chicken in the pan. Fry over a high heat for 1 minute, then spoon the onion and spice mix over the chicken, pressing it into the meat with the back of a spoon. Remove from the heat and cover (use foil if you don't have a lid for the pan). Cook in the oven for 20 minutes.

To serve

Divide the chicken and vegetables between 2 plates and serve immediately.

⚡ UPCYCLE Because the spices permeate the chicken overnight, this is even better enjoyed the next day. Simply spread a wholemeal wrap with Chilli Creamed Corn (see page 176), and fill with cherry tomatoes and a handful of baby leaves along with some diced chicken.

turmeric chicken skewers

Serves: 2
Preparation time: 5 minutes
Cooking time: 10 minutes
Wheat free, Gluten free
Preheat grill to high, and place a non-stick baking tray under it

'Meat on a stick' is ever-popular at street stalls all over South East Asia. You can use metal or wooden skewers. If using wooden skewers, soak them in water just before using them.

1 heaped teaspoon turmeric
¼ teaspoon chilli powder
2 tablespoons lemon juice
1 garlic clove, peeled and crushed
50ml low-fat natural yoghurt

2 free-range chicken breast, skinned and cut into bite-sized pieces

4 skewers, at least 20cm long

Make the marinade by mixing together the turmeric, chilli powder, lemon juice, garlic and yoghurt in a large mixing bowl.

Coat the chicken in the marinade.

Thread the chicken pieces onto the skewers and place on the hot baking tray, pouring over some of the remaining marinade and discarding any excess. Place the tray under the grill and cook, turning the skewers every 2 minutes or so to ensure even cooking.

TIP This recipe is equally delicious with salmon and other firm-textured fish, or peeled king prawns – just adjust the cooking times.

UPCYCLE Combine the cold Turmeric Chicken Skewers with some Barley Couscous Tabbouleh (see page 132), and add freshly chopped cucumber and cooked beetroot along with a handful of flat-leaf parsley for a stunning light lunch.

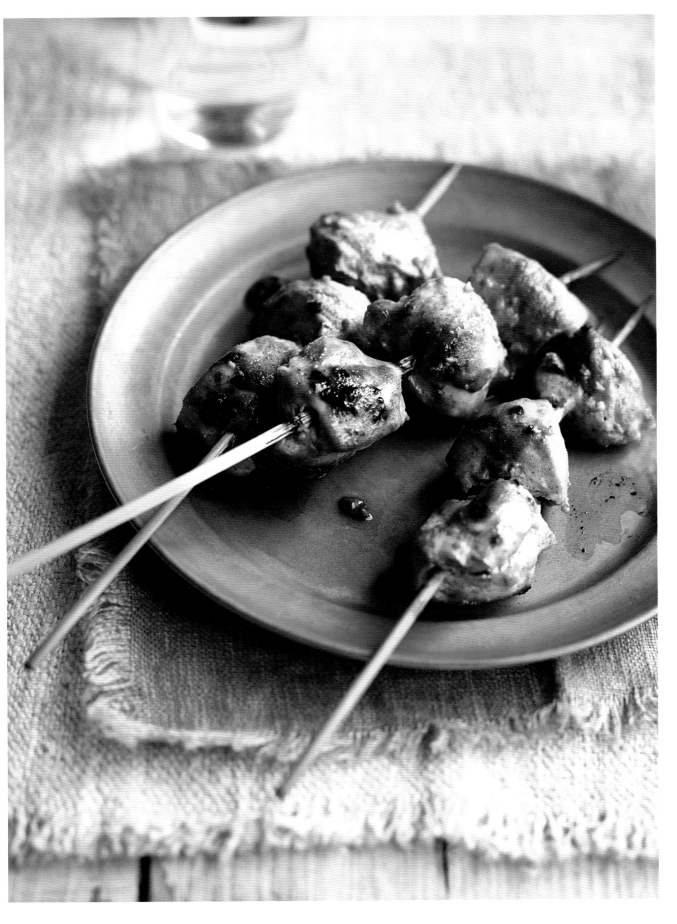

If you've ever been lucky enough to visit Jamaica, you can't have failed to taste their famous jerk seasoning. This chicken recipe, with its kick of chilli and garlic, the zing of ginger and the exotic flavour of allspice, will take you back to the Caribbean.

jerk chicken

Serves: 2
Preparation time: 15 minutes
Cooking time: 20 minutes
Wheat free, Gluten free, Dairy free
Preheat oven to 200°/400°F/Gas mark 6, and place a baking tray inside

1 large spring onion, trimmed and chopped
3cm piece fresh ginger, peeled and chopped
1 large garlic clove, peeled and chopped
1 red chilli, deseeded and chopped
2 teaspoons olive oil
½ teaspoon ground allspice
1 teaspoon chopped fresh thyme
1 tablespoon honey
1 tablespoon tamari soy sauce

2 free-range chicken breasts, skin removed

To serve
Lime wedges

To make the marinade, blend together the spring onion, ginger, garlic, chilli, olive oil, allspice, thyme, honey and soy sauce.

Rub the marinade over the chicken, and place on the hot baking tray.

Cook in the oven for 20 minutes, until the chicken is cooked through and the sauce is bubbling and reduced.

Serve the chicken with the sauce spooned over each breast, and garnish with a lime wedge. Serve immediately.

TIP The spice rub also works well on fish and tofu.

⚡ UPCYCLE The quantities given here make more spice mix than you will need for a meal for two, so you can use it up by making extra chicken. The next day, dice up the chicken and mix it with some chopped mango, diced tomatoes, red onion, coriander and lime juice for a tasty salad.

steak with peppercorn sauce

Peppercorn sauce doesn't need to be loaded with saturated fats. A reduction of wine with added crème fraîche is enough to make the creamiest sauce, perfect for spooning over a simply cooked steak.

Serves: 2
Preparation time: 10 minutes
Cooking time: 10 minutes
Wheat free, Gluten free

2 x 150g fillet steaks
1 teaspoon groundnut oil
Freshly ground black pepper

Sprinkle black pepper and oil over both sides of each steak.

Heat a heavy-based non-stick frying pan over a high heat. Place the steaks down, and leave to cook – without moving – for 2 minutes. Flip them over and cook without moving for a further minute. At this point, gently cut through the steak to ensure it is cooked to your liking; if you prefer it more well done then leave to cook for another minute.

Take the steaks out of the pan and leave them to sit on a wooden board or warmed plate.

50ml red wine
50ml beef or vegetable stock

Pour the red wine and stock into the pan and bring to the boil. Leave to bubble for a couple of minutes until reduced by about a third.

1 teaspoon freshly ground black pepper

Stir in the black pepper.

2 tablespoons half-fat crème fraîche

Take the sauce off the heat and gently mix in the crème fraîche, stirring until fully combined.

To serve
Large handful watercress

Place the steaks on warmed serving plates and spoon over the peppercorn sauce. Serve alongside the watercress.

TIP For a lighter taste, use white wine with pink peppercorns. If you don't have wine you can use whisky instead – just reduce the quantity by half.

 UPCYCLE Spread toasted spelt bread with cream cheese, then top with shredded radish and leftover slices of beef.

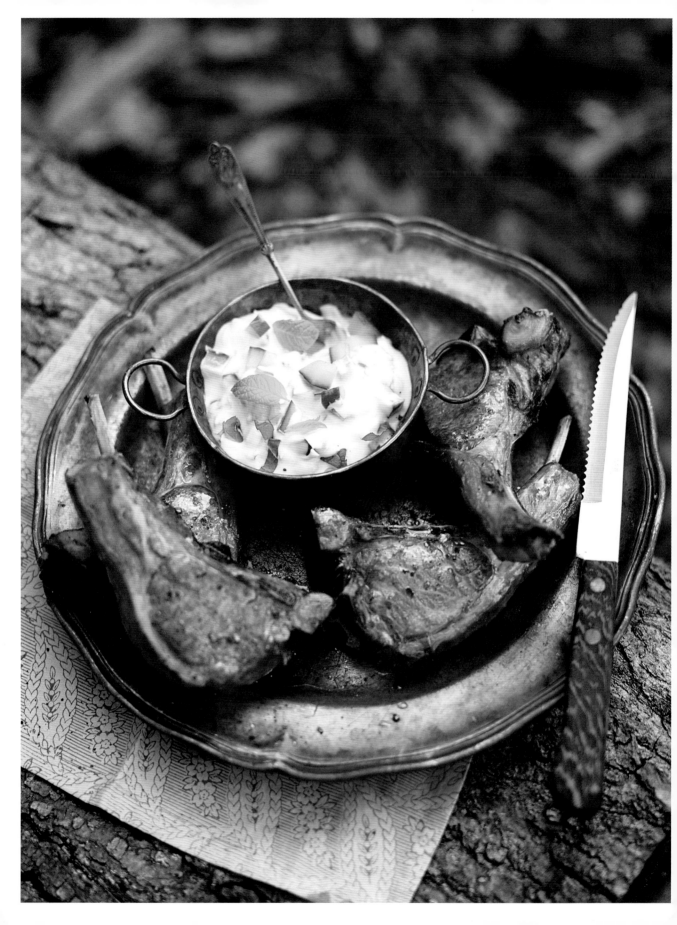

grilled lamb cutlets with mint raita

Little lamb cutlets grilled and served alongside a refreshing mint yoghurt are a favourite in my house – and they take minutes to cook.

Serves: 2
Preparation time: 10 minutes
Cooking time: 6 minutes
Wheat free, Gluten free
Preheat grill to high

3 tablespoons low-fat natural yoghurt
¼ cucumber, peeled, deseeded and roughly chopped
½ garlic clove, crushed
1 tablespoon chopped fresh mint

4 lamb cutlets, at room temperature

To serve

First, make the raita. In a bowl, mix the yoghurt, cucumber, garlic and mint, stirring gently so as not to break up the cucumber. Leave to one side for a few minutes, to allow the flavours to develop.

Meanwhile, cook the lamb. For presentation purposes, use your knife to scrape away any flesh on the exposed bones, then wipe the bones clean using a kitchen paper.

Place the trimmed cutlets under the hot grill for 2–3 minutes on each side (for medium-rare). Remove from the grill and cover with foil for 5 minutes before serving.

Place the lamb chops on a serving plate with the raita on the side. Eat immediately.

TIP Lamb chops also work wonderfully with Mint Pesto (see page 97), either as an accompanying sauce or as a marinade.

blue cheese burgers

Serves: 2
Preparation time: 20 minutes (including chilling time)
Cooking time: 10 minutes
Wheat free, Gluten free

A 'cheeseburger' of sorts, except the lettuce encases the meat, and the cheese is hidden inside. The result is a fantastic combination of textures – a delicious crunch to start with, followed by a delectable cheese sauce that oozes out with every bite of the burger.

40g blue cheese

In a small bowl, break up the blue cheese and roll into 4 balls. Return them to the fridge.

250g lean minced beef
10g flat-leaf parsley, finely chopped
Freshly ground black pepper

In a large bowl, mix together the beef, parsley and black pepper. Divide the mixture into 4 and roll into small balls.

With your thumb, make a deep well in the centre of each ball, into which pop a chilled cheese ball. Cover with the meat to create a complete seal, so that no cheese is visible. Repeat with the others.

Place the balls in the fridge for 10 minutes to firm up before cooking.

1 tablespoon groundnut oil

Heat the oil in a non-stick frying pan over a high heat, and quickly brown the burgers – about 1 minute per side. Then reduce the heat and cook them for a further 3 minutes on each side.

To serve
4 little gem or iceberg lettuce leaves
Small handful cherry tomatoes, halved

Place one meatball in the middle of each lettuce leaf and wrap the leaf around it. Transfer to warmed serving plates and eat immediately with the tomatoes.

TIP I love the tang of blue cheese, but this recipe works just as well with a semi-hard goat's cheese. If your choice of cheese doesn't easily form into balls, just cut it into small cubes and stuff the meatballs as per above.

UPCYCLE Try using the meatballs as a topping for a steaming baked potato – just crumble it over the top or mash the two together. Top with a dollop of soured cream or plain yoghurt for a cooling finish.

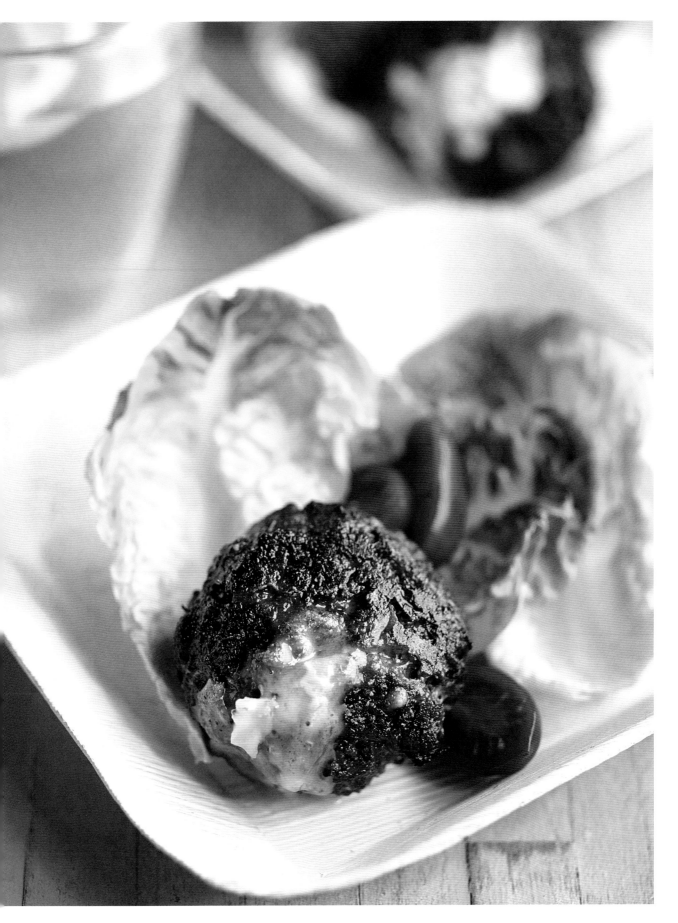

beef & broccoli in oyster sauce

Serves: 2
Preparation time: 10 minutes
Cooking time: 10 minutes
Wheat free, Gluten free, Dairy free

Ready in minutes, this is a dish that really packs a punch with garlic, ginger and chilli – as well as supplying you with antioxidants. All the different flavours and textures are brought together in a sticky oyster sauce. Sublime!

1 tablespoon groundnut oil

Heat the oil in a seasoned wok or large non-stick pan over a high heat.

2 tablespoons good-quality oyster sauce
200g beef fillet, thinly sliced

Put the oyster sauce and beef in a bowl together so they are well mixed.

200g broccoli, cut into florets
1 garlic clove, thinly sliced
5cm piece fresh ginger, peeled and finely chopped
½ red chilli, deseeded and finely chopped

Add the broccoli, garlic, ginger and chilli to the pan, and cook, stirring, for 2 minutes.

125ml water

Add the oyster sauce, beef and water, bring to the boil, and leave to bubble on a high heat for 2 minutes. Reduce the sauce down to about half (it should be very sticky and the beef very tender).

2 spring onions, trimmed and roughly chopped

Add the spring onions, and stir gently over a high heat for another minute.

To serve

Serve in bowls and eat immediately.

TIP Beef, broccoli and oyster sauce are a match made in heaven, but this dish is equally delicious with mushrooms. Simply replace the broccoli with 150g finely sliced portobello mushrooms and continue as above.

⤵ UPCYCLE Any leftovers can be stirred through an equal amount of barley couscous and finish with a good squeeze of lemon juice.

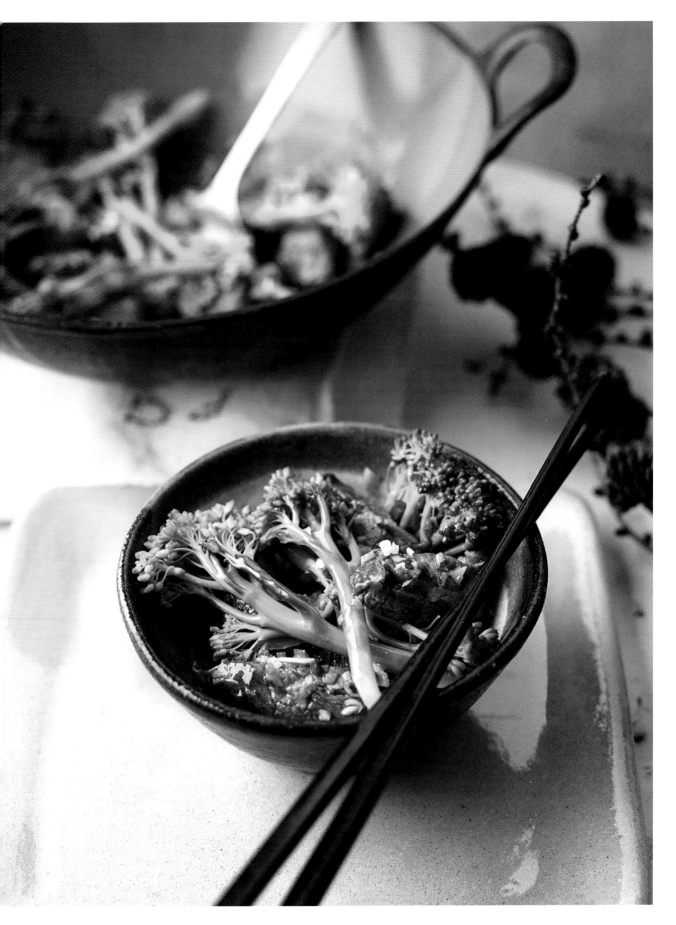

carb sides

IT can be a challenge balancing healthy eating with a busy life. Keeping a few key principles in mind, however, will transform healthy eating into a life-long habit. Eating in the correct proportions is fundamental, and here you should follow the Rule of Palm (see page 8), making sure your breakfast, lunch and dinner combine a good balance of protein and carbohydrates. The recipes in the pages that follow offer tempting and delicious ideas for sides rich in carbohydrates. For a healthy and balanced diet, the aim should be to consume more complex carbohydrates: ingredients such as brown rice, potatoes with their skin on, corn and barley release their energy slowly and can really put the extra 'oomph' into comfort food.

These carb sides have been chosen for their versatility. They are easy to adapt to all kinds of meals and will suit whatever the occasion demands. As well as providing slow and steady levels of energy, the sides include other essential dietary elements, such as good fats, nutrition-rich herbs and leafy greens, and the occasional dash of calcium-dense dairy. I hope that once you have tried these easy and tasty recipes, incorporating more of the right carbs on to your plate will become second nature.

barley couscous tabbouleh

Serves: 2
Preparation time: 10 minutes
Cooking time: 10 minutes
Wheat free, Dairy free, Vegetarian

For our version of tabbouleh, we've substituted barley couscous for the traditional bulgur wheat. The barley gives this dish a nuttier, more wholesome taste and texture.

2 teaspoons olive oil
1 red onion, finely diced
1 garlic clove, finely chopped

Place the oil in a small pan over a low heat. Add the onion and garlic, stir and then cover. Sweat for about 5–7 minutes, until soft.

1 teaspoon ground cumin

Add the cumin to the onion mix and stir thoroughly. Leave to cook for 2 minutes.

80g barley couscous
160ml hot vegetable stock

Place the couscous in a large salad bowl, add the onion mix and pour over the hot stock. Cover with cling film and leave for 5–10 minutes so that the liquid absorbs.

Small handful fresh parsley, finely chopped
Small handful fresh mint, finely chopped
2 spring onions, white parts only, finely sliced

Fluff up the couscous with a fork, then mix through the parsley, mint and spring onion, so that they are evenly incorporated.

¼ cucumber, deseeded and cut into small dice
2 tomatoes, quartered, deseeded and diced

Stir the cucumber and tomatoes into the couscous mix.

To serve
1 tablespoon olive oil
Juice of ½ lemon
Freshly ground black pepper

In a small bowl, mix the olive oil, lemon juice and black pepper. Drizzle over the couscous and serve.

TIP To add a bit of kick to the tabbouleh, add ½ small red chilli, deseeded and finely chopped, and the zest of ½ lemon (added with the herbs).

UPCYCLE Fry slices of halloumi in a griddle pan then toss with a portion of tabbouleh to make a substantial and well-balanced lunch.

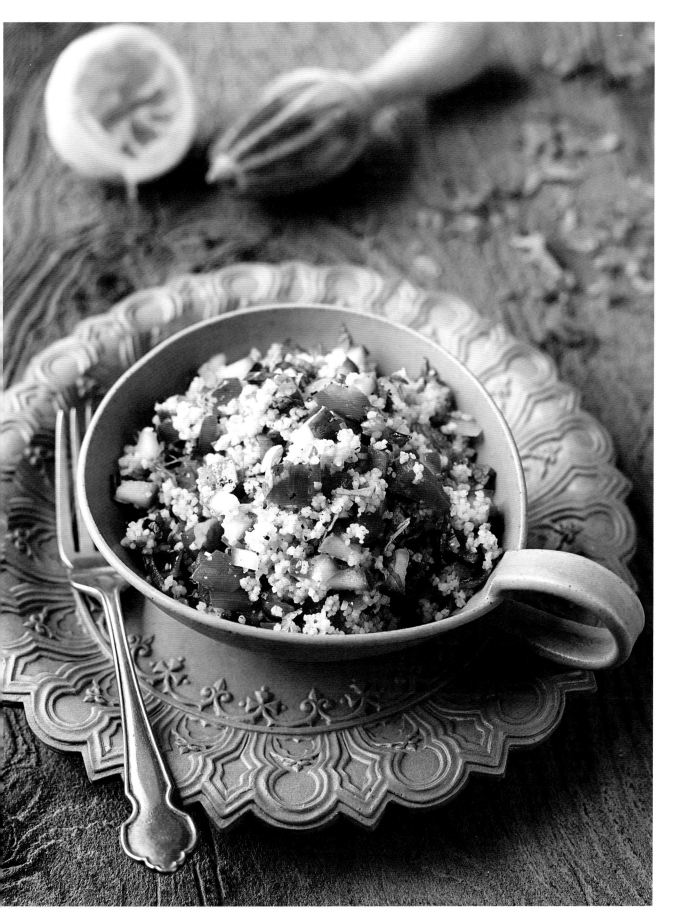

coconut potatoes

Serves: 2
Preparation time: 10 minutes
Cooking time: 25 minutes
Wheat free, Gluten free, Dairy free, Vegetarian

There is something so moreish about potatoes that are cooked in fragrant spices and creamy coconut milk. Try this alongside a piece of simply grilled fish, transforming it into the perfect comfort food.

2 teaspoons groundnut oil
1 small red onion, peeled and finely diced
1 garlic clove, peeled and finely diced
3cm piece of fresh ginger, peeled and finely diced

Heat the oil, onion, garlic and ginger in a medium non-stick saucepan. Cook for 5 minutes over a medium heat, stirring occasionally.

½ large green chilli, deseeded
½ tablespoon coriander seeds, crushed

Add the chilli and coriander seeds, and stir. Leave to cook for a further minute.

225ml half-fat coconut milk
½ cinnamon stick, lightly crushed
2 cardamom pods, lightly crushed

Add the coconut milk, cinnamon stick and cardamom pods. Stir well and bring to the boil.

10 baby potatoes, scrubbed

Add the potatoes and mix well, then top up with water if necessary – you want the potatoes to be just covered by the liquid. Bring to the boil again, then lower the heat and simmer gently for about 15 minutes, or until the potatoes are soft.

Drain the potatoes, keeping the liquid. Sieve the liquid, removing the chilli, cinnamon stick and cardamom pods, then add the remaining liquid back to the potatoes. I sometimes like to use a fork to gently crush the potatoes, breaking them up as they soak up the broth.

To serve
Lime wedges

Add a squeeze of lime juice and serve immediately.

UPCYCLE If you have any leftover potatoes, turn them into a substantial meal by adding cooked prawns, lightly cooked green beans or asparagus, shredded spinach leaves and heat through.

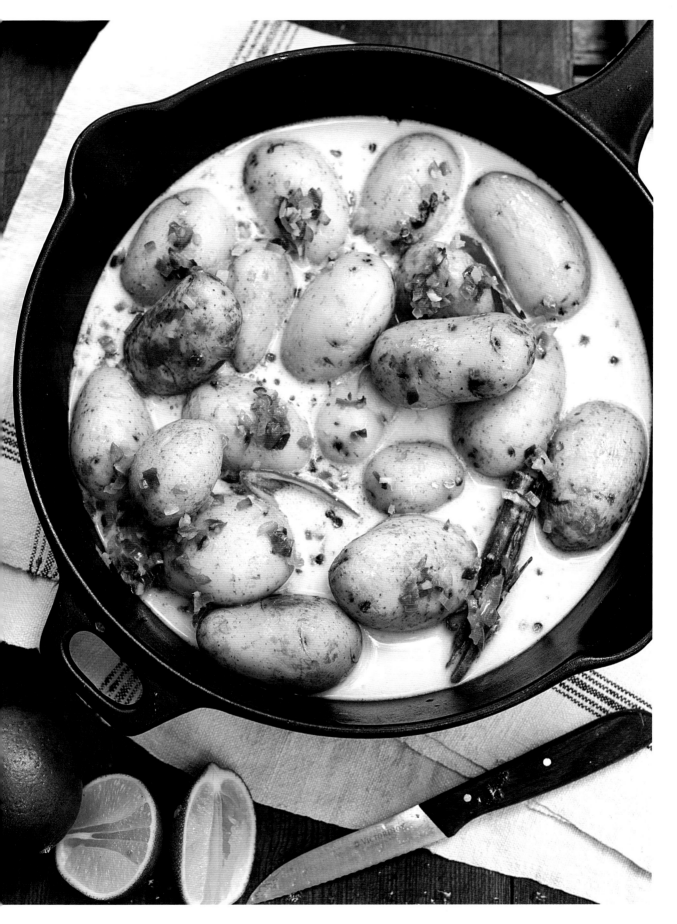

butter bean, garlic & rosemary mash

This recipe started life as a high-protein topping for pies, but has become a favourite in its own right – not just because it is delicious, but also because it is a nutritious alternative to mashed potatoes.

Serves: 2
Preparation time: 20 minutes
Cooking time: 10 minutes
Wheat free, Gluten free, Dairy free, Vegetarian

3 garlic cloves, peeled
1 tablespoon olive oil

Place the whole garlic cloves and the oil in a non-stick frying pan and cook over a medium heat until they become soft – about 5 minutes. Once soft, place in a small bowl and mash to a paste.

1 teaspoon finely chopped fresh rosemary leaves

Add the rosemary and continue mashing until the ingredients are well combined.

200g tin butter beans, drained and rinsed
1 tablespoon vegetable stock

While the garlic is sweating, bring the butter beans up to boil in a pan of water for 3 minutes. Drain.

In a shallow bowl, mash the butter beans and stock together with a fork, until it has reached your preferred consistency. Add the garlic and rosemary paste and stir to combine thoroughly.

To serve
Freshly ground black pepper

Spoon into a warmed serving dish, sprinkle with black pepper, and serve immediately.

TIP I love the creamy texture of butter beans, but you can substitute other tinned pulses such as borlotti beans, pinto beans, or even chickpeas.

UPCYCLE Make a scrumptious dip or sandwich spread by adding very finely chopped anchovies and a splash of milk to the mash. Stir together well.

thyme & oregano baked chips

Serves: 2
Preparation time: 5 minutes
Cooking time: 15 minutes
Wheat free, Gluten free, Dairy Free, Vegetarian
Preheat oven to 200°C/400°F/Gas mark 6, and place a non-stick baking tray inside

A great alternative to supermarket-bought oven chips. They take less time to cook, and keeping the skins on provides a great source of fibre as well as giving a deep, earthy flavour.

2 medium-sized potatoes, cut into 2cm cubes
1 tablespoon olive oil
1 teaspoon dried oregano
1 teaspoon dried thyme

To serve
Freshly ground black pepper

Rub the potato cubes with oil, dried oregano and thyme.

Place on the hot baking tray and bake for about 15 minutes, shaking the tray after about 10 minutes.

Season with a little black pepper and serve immediately.

UPCYCLE Combine leftover potatoes with slices of grilled halloumi and some baby spinach or rocket, and fill a wholemeal pitta bread.

137

bombay potatoes

This is a fantastic way to prepare baby new potatoes; the vibrant spices will give your tastebuds a wake-up call.

Serves: 2
Preparation time: 5 minutes
Cooking time: 20 minutes
Wheat free, Gluten free, Dairy free, Vegetarian

250g baby new potatoes, halved

1 tablespoon groundnut oil
1 teaspoon cumin seeds
1 teaspoon mustard seeds
1 teaspoon fennel seeds
1 teaspoon turmeric

To serve
Small handful fresh coriander, finely chopped

Cook the potatoes in a pan of boiling water for 10–15 minutes until tender.

While the potatoes are cooking, heat the oil in a medium non-stick pan over a medium heat, and add all of the spices. Stir thoroughly to coat them with oil; the spices will crackle and pop but don't worry. Leave to cook for 2–3 minutes, stirring frequently.

Drain the potatoes and add them straight to the pan with the spices. Stir well, so that the spices coat the potatoes evenly.

Sprinkle with the coriander and serve immediately.

🔁 UPCYCLE For a quick, tasty supper, cut some firm tofu into bite-sized cubes, stir-fry in a teaspoon of oil, and mix through with the leftover potatoes. Add a handful of cherry tomatoes and some chopped fresh spinach.

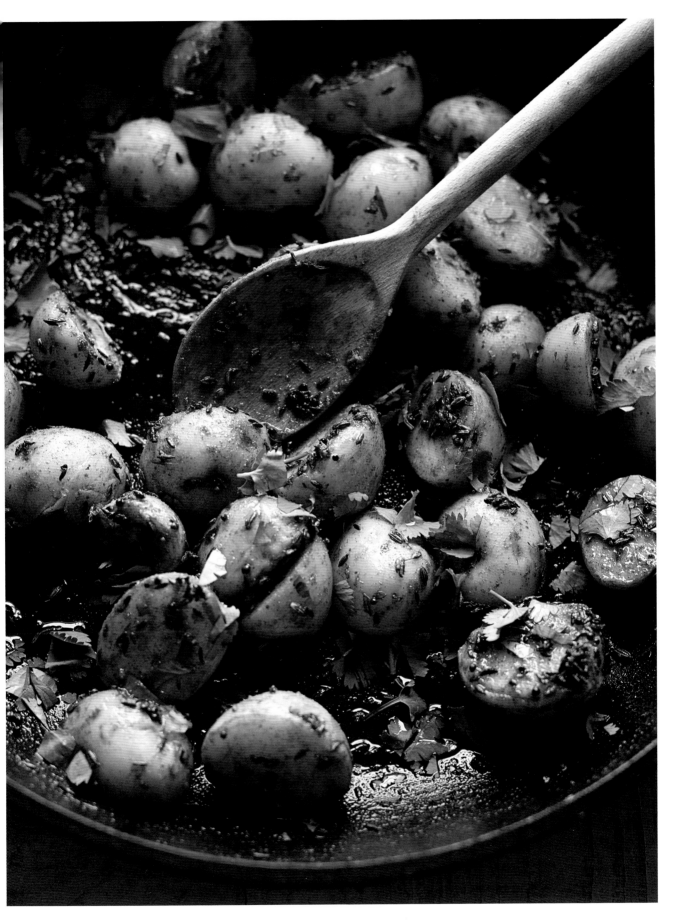

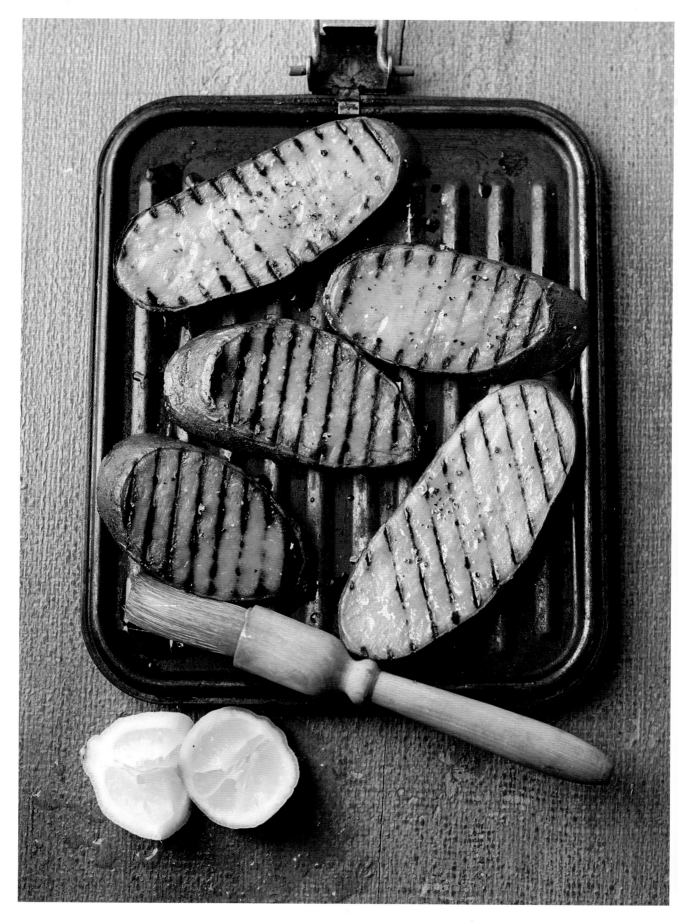

garlic-grilled sweet potatoes

Serves: 2
Preparation time: 5 minutes
Cooking time: 15 minutes
Wheat free, Gluten free, Dairy free, Vegetarian

This is a simple but striking way to cook sweet potatoes. In summer, I like to grill these on the barbecue, giving them a deep, smoky flavour.

1 tablespoon olive oil
1 garlic clove, thinly sliced

1 large sweet potato, scrubbed and cut lengthways into 2cm thick slices

To serve
Lemon wedges
Freshly ground black pepper

First prepare the garlic oil. Place the oil and the garlic in a small saucepan over a low heat, so that the oil and the garlic warm through together. As soon as the garlic starts to sizzle, take the pan off the heat and set aside.

Fill a large pan with water and bring to the boil. Add the sweet potato slices, reduce the heat and leave to simmer for about 6 minutes – a sharp knife should just be able to pierce the centre. Drain the potatoes, taking care not to break the slices, and lay on a flat surface.

Lightly brush the top of each slice with the garlic-infused oil.

Heat a griddle pan over a medium–high heat.

Place the potato slices in the hot griddle pan and cook for 2 minutes. Turn them over, lightly brush the other side with the oil, and cook for 2 more minutes.

Serve immediately, with a squeeze of lemon juice over each slice, and a sprinkling of black pepper.

TIP Infusing olive oil with flavours is a simple and quick way to liven up a dish – try it also with slices of fresh chilli, some citrus rind, or a sprig of rosemary. The trick is to place the flavours in the oil before you heat it through, and to remove the oil from the heat before it starts to spit.

UPCYCLE These sweet potatoes make a great addition to any green salad. Add some blue cheese, a handful of walnuts, and a simple olive oil and honey dressing, and you've got lunch ready in minutes.

algerian wedding rice

In Algeria, this dish is served at weddings and makes great use of the abundance of dried fruit and nuts. Traditionally a slow-cooked rice dish; we've simplified the process.

Serves: 2
Preparation time: 10 minutes
Cooking time: 30 minutes
Wheat free, Gluten free, Dairy free, Vegetarian

80g quick-cook brown rice
160ml vegetable stock or water

Place the rice and vegetable stock or water in a saucepan and bring to the boil. Once it's boiling, reduce the heat so that it simmers, then cover tightly and cook for 20–25 minutes, or according to packet instructions, until tender. Drain.

2 teaspoons olive oil
2 spring onions, trimmed and finely sliced

Place the olive oil and spring onions in a small non-stick pan and heat for a couple of minutes.

20g ready-to-eat dried apricots, roughly chopped into small bite-sized pieces
15g almonds, roughly chopped
15g pine nuts

Add the remaining ingredients to the pan. Add the cooked, drained rice and stir for a couple of minutes until well mixed.

To serve
Freshly ground black pepper

Serve with a sprinkling of black pepper on top.

UPCYCLE Add some chopped fresh mango and cucumber to the rice and toss together with mixed leaves to make a delicious rice salad.

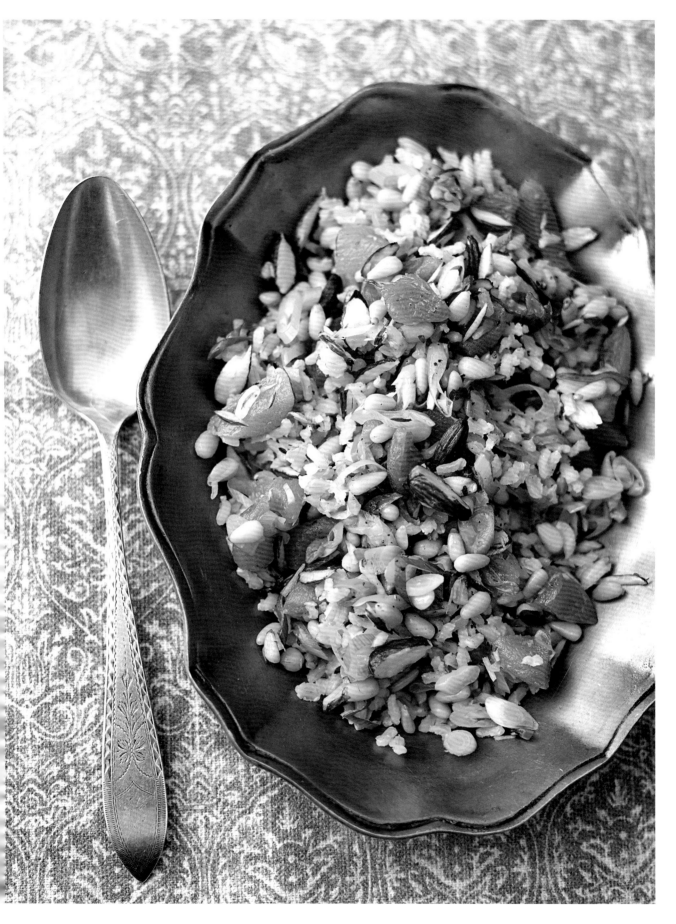

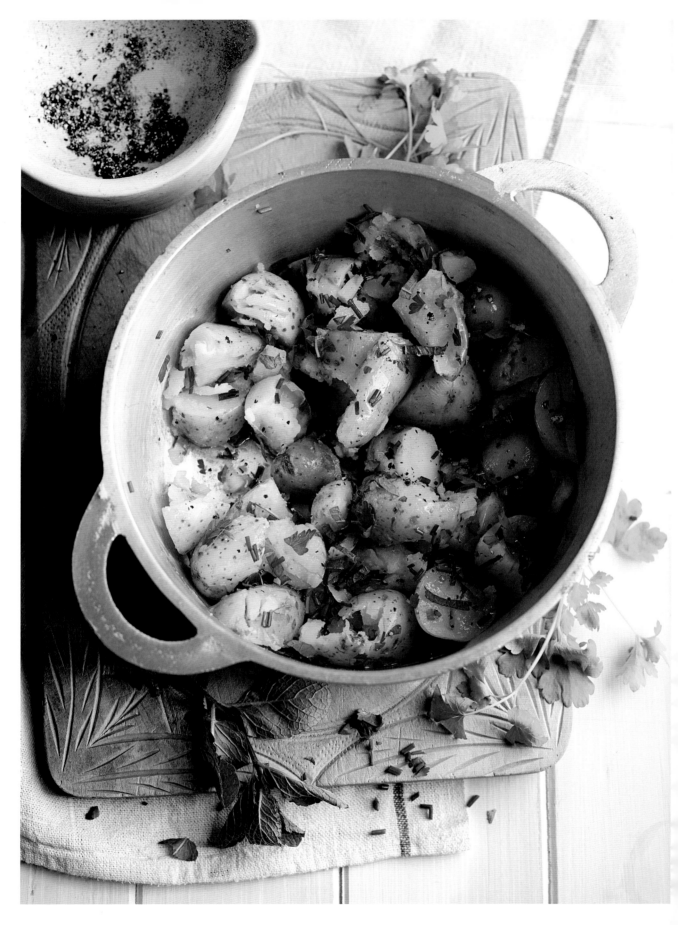

herby smashed new potatoes

Serves: 2
Preparation time: 5 minutes
Cooking time: 15 minutes
Wheat free, Gluten free, Dairy free, Vegetarian

Early summer brings an abundance of new potatoes. These are best enjoyed simply tossed with fresh herbs, which enhance their natural sweetness.

200g new potatoes, scrubbed and cut in half

Small handful fresh parsley, finely chopped
Small handful fresh mint, finely chopped
Few fresh chives, finely chopped
1 tablespoon olive oil
Freshly ground black pepper

Put the potatoes in a large pan of boiling water and cook at a steady boil until a fork easily pierces them – about 12 minutes.

Meanwhile, in a small bowl mix the herbs, olive oil and black pepper.

Drain the potatoes and return to the pan. Add the herb mixture and stir through, then partially mash the potatoes using either the back of a wooden spoon or a potato masher. You don't want to completely mash the potatoes, just to break them up, so that the herbs are crushed into them.

To serve

Serve immediately in a warmed heavy dish.

UPCYCLE Heat the leftover potatoes in a non-stick frying pan over a medium heat, then add 2 beaten eggs along with chopped fresh herbs. Allow to cook over a low heat for 3 minutes, grate over Parmesan, then place under a hot grill until bubbling and golden.

coconut rice

Cooking rice in coconut milk makes it wonderfully fragrant and the brown basmati adds extra fibre and nuttiness.

Serves: 2
Preparation time: 5 minutes
Cooking time: 30 minutes
Wheat free, Gluten free, Dairy free, Vegetarian

1 tablespoon groundnut or coconut oil
1 garlic clove, peeled and finely sliced

80g quick-cook brown basmati rice
250ml half-fat coconut milk
80ml water

1 small handful coconut flakes

To serve
Juice of ½ lime

Place the oil and garlic in a small pan over a low heat.

When the garlic starts to sizzle, add the rice, and stir to mix. Add the coconut milk and water, stir well, and bring to the boil. Then reduce the heat, cover the pan with a tight-fitting lid, and leave to simmer for 25–30 minutes or according to the packet instructions.

Toast the coconut flakes in a small non-stick frying pan over a high heat, until just browned. While still warm, stir through the cooked rice.

Fluff up the rice with a fork, spoon it into a serving dish, squeeze over the lime juice and serve immediately.

TIP The trick with cooking rice in a pan is to ensure that the lid fits really tightly. One easy way to create a complete seal is to cut a piece of parchment paper into a round roughly the shape of your pan, and place this on the surface of the rice before fitting the lid; this will ensure the rice cooks perfectly.

UPCYCLE Any leftover coconut rice will make wonderful fried rice the next day. Heat some oil in a wok and simply fry some grated ginger and chopped spring onions, add chopped vegetables of your choice, then stir in the rice, tamari soy sauce and a squeeze of lime. Top with a poached egg for a lovely supper dish.

creamy herbed polenta

Serves: 2
Preparation time: 5 minutes
Cooking time: 10 minutes
Wheat free, Vegetarian

Polenta – ground cornmeal – is a staple of northern Italy. The beauty of it is that it can be used as a creamy and comforting alternative to pasta or mashed potatoes.

200ml vegetable stock 200ml water	Place the stock and water in a large pan and bring to the boil.
100g fine polenta	Reduce the heat so that the liquid is simmering, then pour in the polenta in a steady stream, stirring constantly with a wooden spoon or whisk until all of the polenta has been added.
40g Parmesan cheese, finely grated 1 tablespoon finely chopped fresh tarragon	Keep stirring until all of the liquid has been absorbed – about a minute or so – before adding the Parmesan and tarragon. Allow it to bubble for a further minute, stirring constantly.
To serve	Pour the creamy polenta mix into a warmed bowl and serve immediately.

TIP A great alternative to the Parmesan cheese is goat's cheese.

UPCYCLE Polenta firms up once cooled, and can be cut into thick wedges, which can be grilled. To make crispy polenta wedges, pour any excess polenta, while still warm, into a shallow non-stick tray, smooth over, and leave to cool for at least an hour. Cut into wedges, brush lightly with olive oil, and place under a hot grill.

stir-fry noodles

Serves: 2
Preparation time: 15 minutes
Cooking time: 10 minutes
Wheat free, Gluten free, Dairy free

I love vermicelli for its moreish melt-in-your mouth quality. You can easily substitute any noodles available, just cook them according to the packet instructions.

80g rice vermicelli noodles

First, prepare the noodles. Soak them in a bowl of just-boiled water for 3 minutes until tender, or according to the packet instructions. Drain and set aside.

2 teaspoons groundnut oil
1 teaspoon sesame oil
1 spring onion, trimmed and thinly sliced
1 garlic clove, peeled and finely sliced
½ red chilli, deseeded and finely chopped
2cm piece fresh ginger, peeled and finely chopped

Heat the oils in a wok or medium non-stick pan over a high heat, then add the spring onion, garlic, chilli and ginger, stirring constantly.

Add the soaked noodles to the wok and toss well.

2 tablespoons tamari soy sauce
2 tablespoons Thai fish sauce
Juice of ½ lime

Add the soy sauce, fish sauce and lime juice and mix well, until all the ingredients are combined and the wok is sizzling.

To serve
1 tablespoon finely chopped fresh coriander
1 spring onion, trimmed and finely chopped

Spoon into serving bowls and sprinkle the coriander and spring onion over the top.

UPCYCLE For a really easy rice noodle salad, mix leftovers with grated carrot, shredded cucumber, and cherry tomato halves. Drizzle with sesame oil and a tablespoon of rice wine vinegar, then top with cooked prawns or shredded cooked chicken.

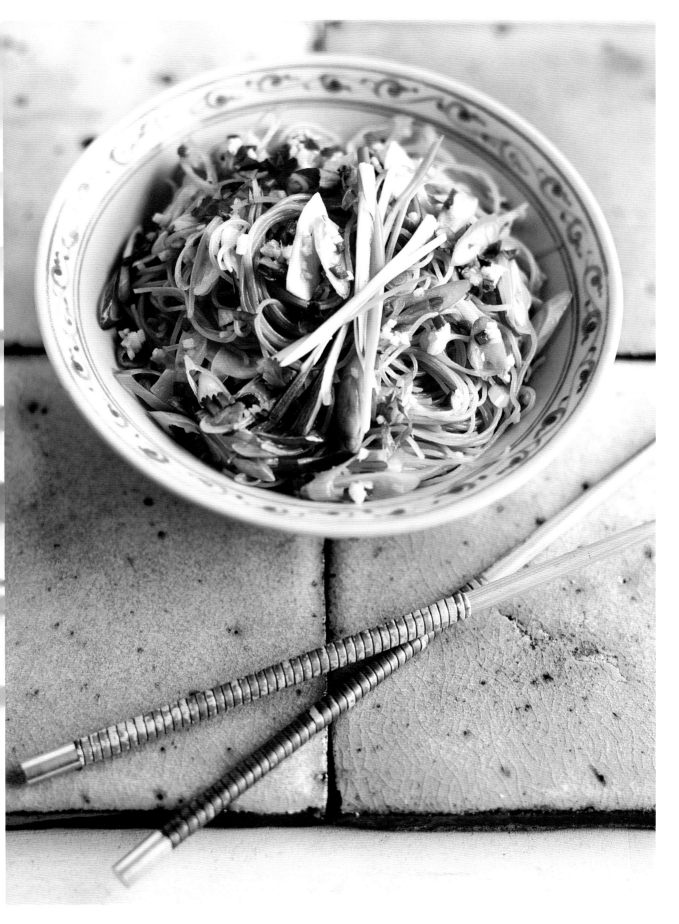

veg sides

EATING a wonderful array of colour is one of The Pure Package's fundamental principles: incorporating a variety of naturally coloured foods into our diet gives our bodies all the vitamins, minerals and antioxidants necessary for radiant health. For brighter eyes, clearer skin and an all-over glow, the delicious vegetable recipes that follow will help your body to be its best.

What I love about cooking with vegetables is the sheer versatility. The added bonus is the nutrients they offer, making up an integral part of a balanced diet. These recipes are designed to be changeable and adaptable: serve them as they appear here – as side dishes to mains – or use them as the basis of stand-alone meals in their own right. Some vegetable dishes are perfect paired with a slice of wholegrain bread or a portion of lean protein. Others are delicious piled high on top of a slice of toasted rye bread that has been spread with cream cheese – a great snack for when you need some extra energy.

However you choose to use the following recipes, you can rest easy knowing that you're introducing more of the rainbow on to your plate.

A versatile dish that will match almost any main brilliantly. Use a variety of carrots if you can – a mixture of purple, yellow and orange will bring colour and goodness to your plate.

balsamic carrots

Serves: 2
Preparation time: 15 minutes
Wheat free, Gluten free, Dairy free, Vegetarian

1 tablespoon olive oil
1 tablespoon balsamic vinegar
½ teaspoon Dijon mustard
Freshly ground black pepper

2 carrots, peeled and sliced very thinly
(use a potato peeler)
1 celery stalk, finely chopped
½ red pepper, deseeded and finely sliced
2 spring onions, trimmed and
finely chopped

To serve

First make the dressing. Combine the olive oil, vinegar, mustard and pepper in a small bowl and whisk with a fork.

Put the carrots, celery, red pepper and spring onions into a large salad bowl and stir to combine. Drizzle the dressing over the vegetables, stir well to combine, and leave to one side for a few minutes for the flavours to infuse.

Serve directly from the salad bowl.

UPCYCLE Any leftover salad can be served on top of rye toast along with crumbled goat's or feta cheese.

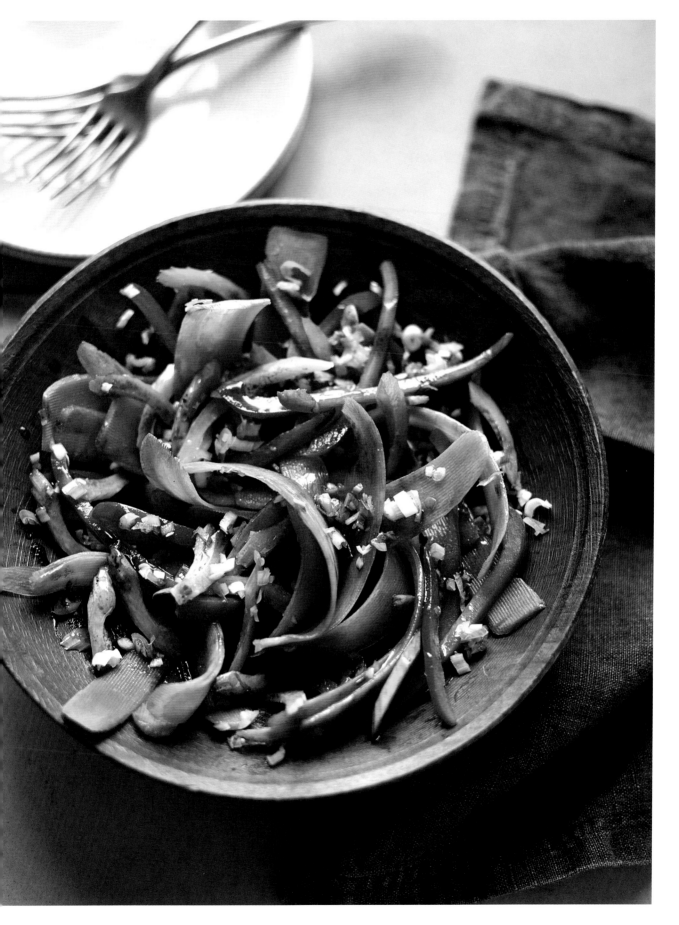

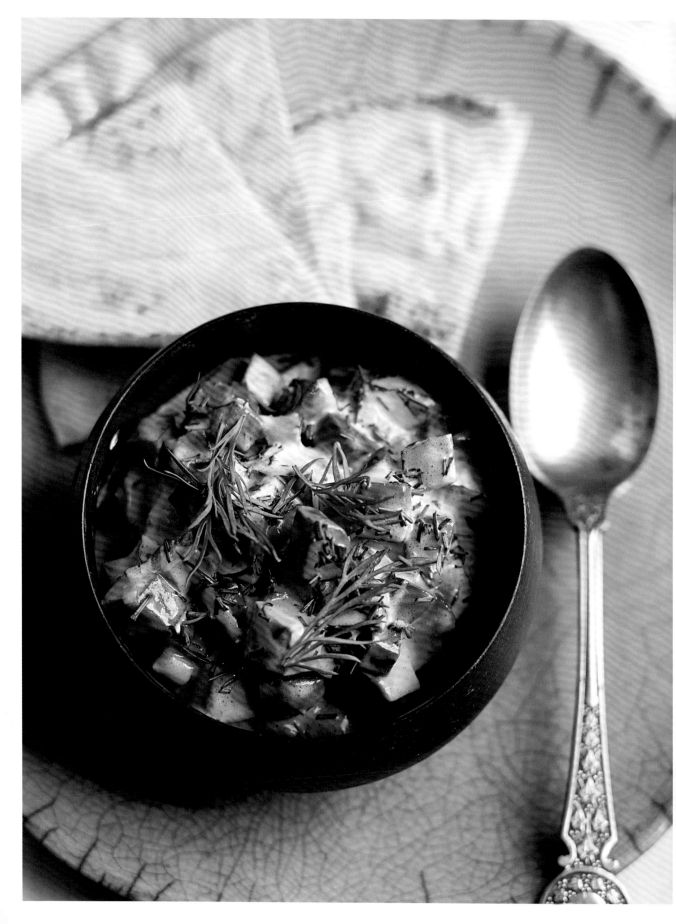

beetroot tzatziki

Serves: 2
Preparation time: 25 minutes, including
10 minutes chilling time
Wheat free, Gluten free, Vegetarian

This sweet yet tangy tzatziki works just as well as a dip as it does nestled up to fish or meat. It's completely moreish so you may find yourself just tucking into the bowl with a spoon!

1 tablespoon olive oil
1 tablespoon wine vinegar (red or white)
100ml goat's milk yoghurt

¼ cucumber, deseeded and finely diced
100g cooked beetroot, finely diced
Small handful fresh mint, finely chopped
Small handful fresh dill, finely chopped

To serve
1 tablespoon finely chopped fresh dill

Mix the oil and vinegar with the yoghurt.

Add the cucumber and beetroot, stir well, then mix in the herbs. Cover and put in the fridge for 15 minutes.

Sprinkle with the dill to serve.

TIP I like to use goat's milk yoghurt for its sharpness but you could easily use sheep's milk yoghurt or Greek-style yoghurt instead.

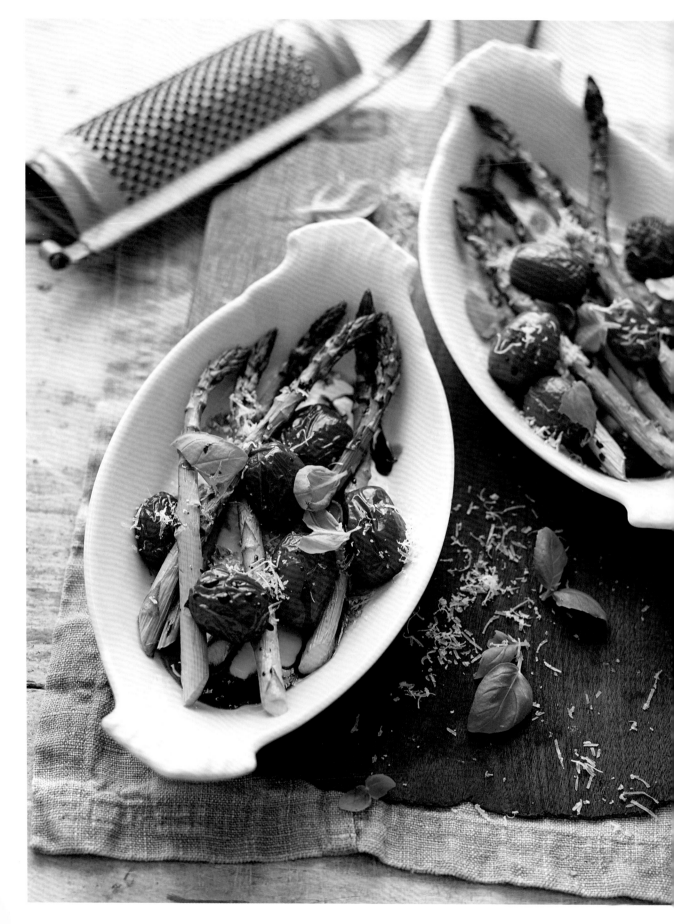

roasted asparagus & baby tomatoes with basil

Roasting the asparagus for a short time preserves its bite while the baby tomatoes provide a lovely sweet and sticky juice. Another effortless dish!

Serves: 2
Preparation time: 5 minutes
Cooking time: 15 minutes
Wheat free, Gluten free, Vegetarian
Preheat oven to 200°C/400°F/Gas mark 6

10 asparagus spears, trimmed
12 cherry tomatoes

1 tablespoon balsamic vinegar

To serve
2 tablespoons finely grated Parmesan cheese
Small handful basil leaves

In 2 small ovenproof dishes, place the asparagus in a single layer and scatter over the tomatoes.

Drizzle the vinegar over the vegetables. Place in the oven for 10–12 minutes (depending on the size of the asparagus spears), or until the asparagus is just tender.

Remove from the oven and sprinkle the Parmesan and basil on top. Allow the cheese to melt into the vegetables slightly before serving.

TIP When asparagus isn't in season, substitute fine green beans and use feta instead of Parmesan cheese.

⬈ UPCYCLE For a more substantial meal, slice up leftover asparagus and add to cooked pasta along with some chopped tomatoes and their juices. Add a spoonful of Basil Pesto (see page 97) and toss to combine. Serve with a little grated Parmesan cheese.

honey & balsamic roasted vegetables

Serves: 2
Preparation time: 10 minutes
Cooking time: 25 minutes
Wheat free, Gluten free, Dairy free, Vegetarian
Preheat oven to 200°C/400°F/Gas mark 6

Roasted vegetables aren't just for winter – this summery side is perfect served alongside simply grilled or barbecued lamb chops or chicken pieces.

1 carrot, peeled
1 courgette
1 red onion, peeled
1 red pepper, deseeded
½ yellow pepper, deseeded
80g broccoli florets
1 plum tomato, quartered
2 garlic cloves, unpeeled and squashed
2 teaspoons olive oil

Chop the carrot, courgette, onion and peppers into bite size pieces the same size (this will ensure even cooking). Place all of the vegetables, tomato, garlic and olive oil into a deep baking tray, and toss to combine. Cover with foil and place in the oven for 15 minutes.

1 tablespoon balsamic vinegar
1 tablespoon honey

In a small bowl or jug, mix together the balsamic vinegar and honey.

Freshly ground black pepper

Remove the tin foil from the tray, add the balsamic and honey mix and stir through. Season with black pepper and return to the oven for 10 minutes, or until the vegetables are cooked.

To serve
Squeeze lemon juice

Season with a squeeze of lemon juice and serve immediately.

TIP In the winter months, replace the courgette, broccoli, peppers and tomatoes with root vegetables such as beetroot, parsnip, sweet potato and add a sprig of rosemary to bring everything together.

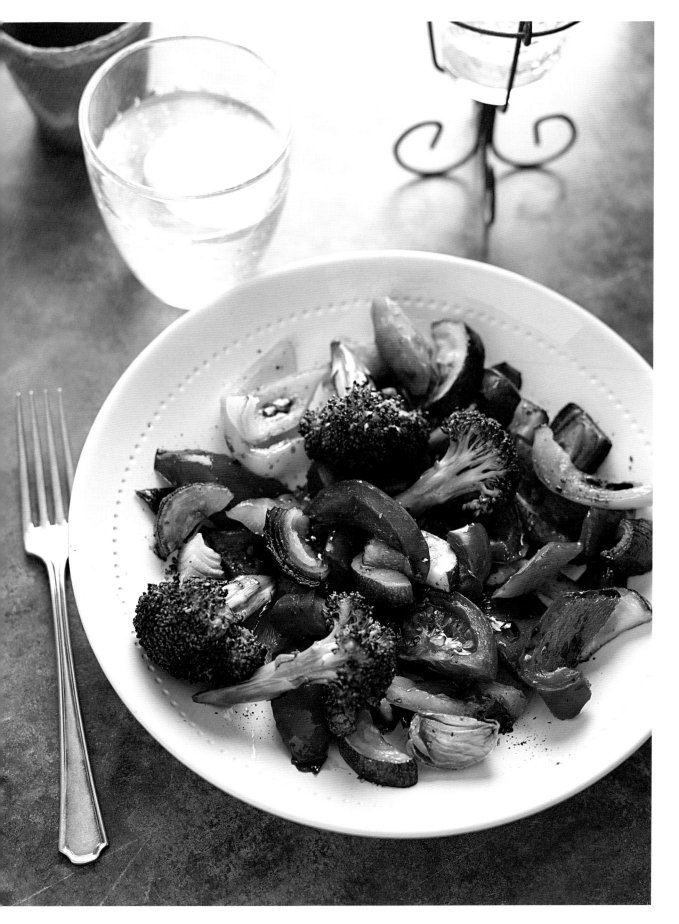

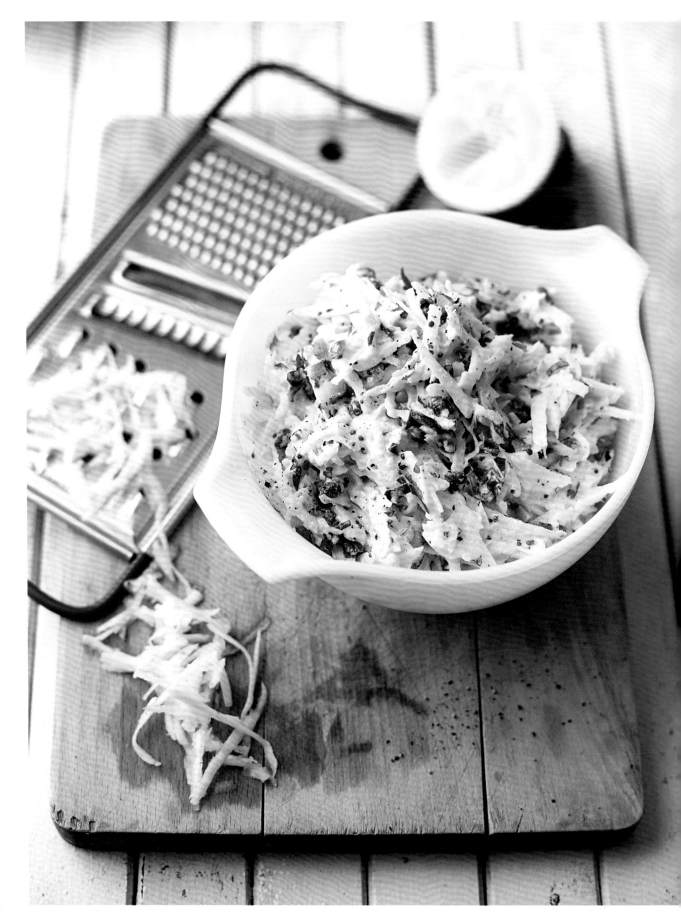

celeriac remoulade

Serves: 2
Preparation time: 10 minutes
Wheat free, Gluten free, Vegetarian

A classic salad of grated celeriac mixed with herbs and mayonnaise is given a twist here. We've added apple for sweetness and the mayonnaise has been replaced with crème fraîche, giving the dish a fresher taste.

50ml half-fat crème fraîche
1 teaspoon wholegrain mustard
Juice of ½ lemon
1 tablespoon capers, rinsed and drained
1 tablespoon cornichons,
roughly chopped

200g celeriac root, peeled and
roughly grated
1 small apple, peeled, cored and grated
1 tablespoon finely chopped
flat-leaf parsley

To serve
Lemon wedges
Freshly ground black pepper

Put the crème fraîche, mustard, lemon juice, capers and cornichons into a jar and shake. Alternatively mix thoroughly in a bowl.

Just before serving, place the celeriac, apple and parsley in a large bowl and add the dressing. Mix well.

Add another squeeze of lemon juice and pepper and serve the remoulade as soon as possible, to prevent discoloration.

UPCYCLE Simply top any leftovers with slices of smoked fish, and serve with a handful of baby greens for a light and summery lunch.

ginger & cabbage stir-fry

Serves: 2
Preparation time: 5 minutes
Cooking time: 10 minutes
Wheat free, Gluten free, Dairy free, Vegetarian

This side dish is bursting with flavour, texture and nutrients. To lock in as much of the goodness of the vegetables as possible, everything needs to be cooked very quickly over a high heat.

2 teaspoons groundnut oil
½ onion, peeled and thinly sliced

1 garlic clove, peeled and finely sliced
5cm piece fresh ginger, peeled and finely chopped or grated

½ head of Savoy cabbage, finely shredded

2 tablespoons tamari soy sauce
1 teaspoon sesame oil
Juice of ½ lime
1 tablespoon finely chopped coriander

To serve
Lime wedges

Heat the oil in a large wok or a non-stick pan over a high heat with the onion and stir-fry for a few minutes.

Add the garlic and ginger, stirring constantly.

After another minute add the cabbage. Keeping the heat high, stir the mixture around in the pan so that everything has equal exposure to the heat. Place the lid on and cook for 5 minutes.

Add the soy sauce and sesame oil, mix well, then add the lime juice and coriander. Give everything one final mix before taking the pan off the heat.

Serve directly onto individual plates, or in a warmed serving bowl, and eat immediately.

UPCYCLE Toss with some cooked rice noodles and sprinkle over crushed peanuts or cashew nuts for a substantial lunch.

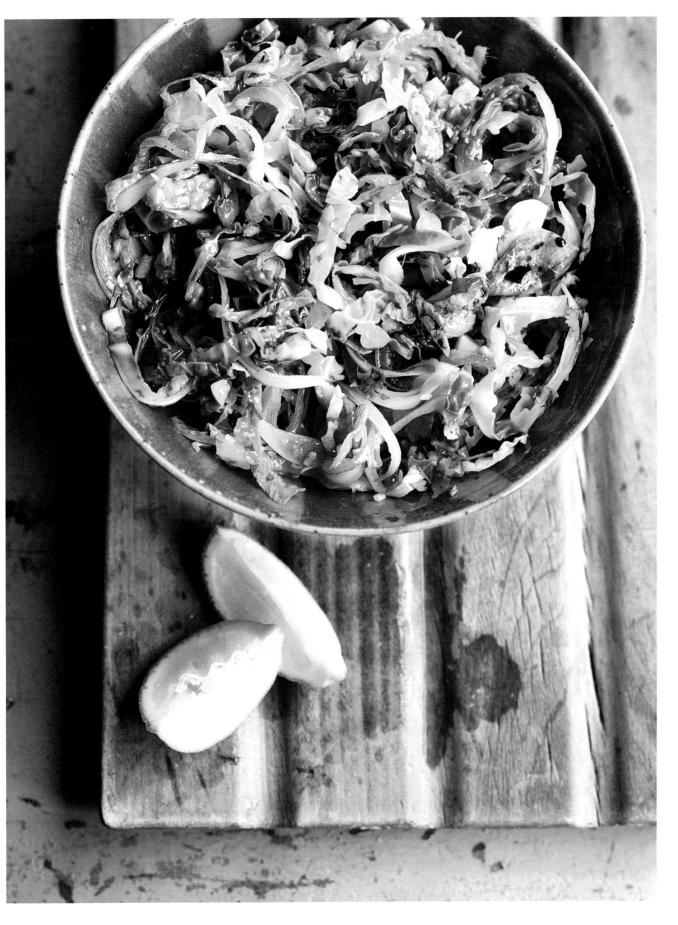

broccoli with garlic & chilli

Serves: 2
Preparation time: 5 minutes
Cooking time: 10 minutes
Wheat free, Gluten free, Dairy free, Vegetarian

The zingy combination of chilli, lemon and garlic always leaves me wanting more. Use both the broccoli florets and stalk to get the most from this super-nutritious vegetable.

2 teaspoons groundnut oil
1 small head broccoli (about 200g), stalks and florets roughly chopped into small pieces

2 tablespoons water
1 garlic clove, peeled and finely chopped
½ red chilli, deseeded and finely chopped

To serve
Juice of ½ lemon
Freshly ground black pepper

Place a deep frying pan or wok over a high heat. When hot, add the oil, swirl to cover the bottom, then add the broccoli. Cover with a lid and stir-fry for 1 minute.

Shake the pan, then remove the lid. Add the water, garlic and chilli. Cover, then shake the pan again (to combine all of the ingredients) and leave for 2 minutes over the high heat, shaking the pan occasionally.

Tip the broccoli into a serving bowl, squeeze the lemon juice directly over it, season with black pepper, and serve while piping hot.

TIP For a real treat, make this with purple sprouting or tender-stem broccoli. You won't need to chop the stalks; just add whole pieces to the pan.

↗ UPCYCLE This makes a great salad base when cooled. Simply toss with a handful of cubed feta cheese, some diced tomatoes and cucumbers, and a handful of chopped hazelnuts. A dash of fresh lemon juice is all you need to dress it.

tomato gratin

This is a fabulously simple dish, which requires next to no preparation. It's best made in summer when you can find flavourful sweet, ripe tomatoes.

Serves: 2
Preparation time: 5 minutes
Cooking time: 30 minutes
Vegetarian
Preheat oven to 170°C/325°F/Gas mark 3

6 tomatoes, sliced
1 tablespoon balsamic vinegar

4 tablespoons fresh wholemeal
(or rye) breadcrumbs

30g hard goat's cheese, grated

To serve
2 tablespoons finely chopped fresh basil

Layer the tomatoes in an 18cm shallow ovenproof dish and pour the balsamic vinegar over the top.

Cover with the breadcrumbs and place in the oven for 25–30 minutes.

Remove from the oven and scatter the cheese on top.

Add the basil when the cheese has melted slightly. Serve while still piping hot.

UPCYCLE When cooled, the tomato gratin can be whizzed in a food processor, transforming it into a tasty dip.

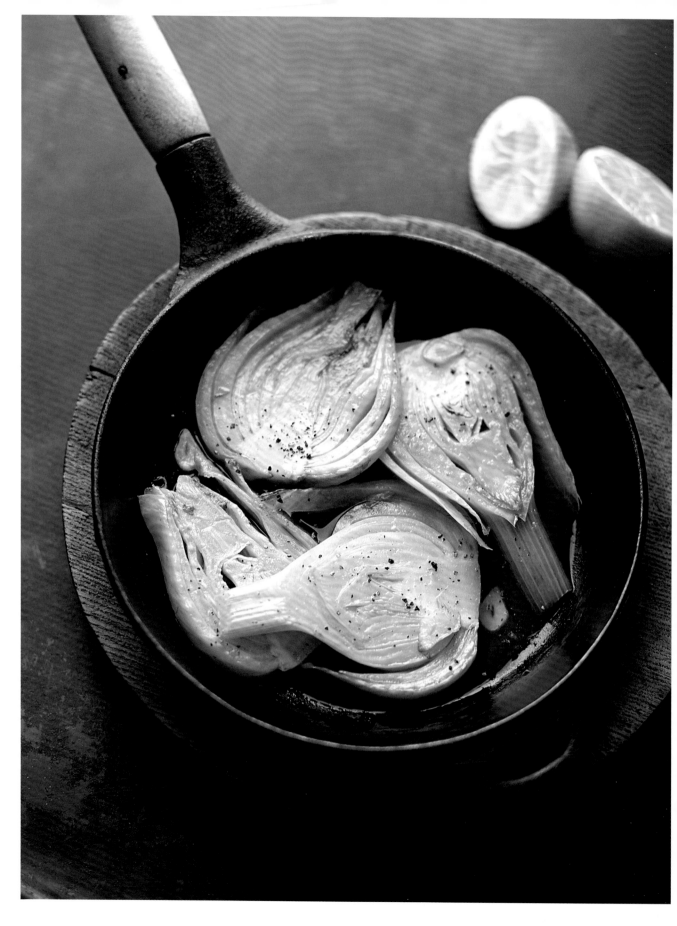

braised fennel

Serves: 2
Preparation time: 5 minutes
Cooking time: 25 minutes
Wheat free, Gluten free, Dairy free, Vegetarian

Fennel is delicious both raw or cooked in any manner of ways, but when braised in wine its aniseed flavour softens considerably.

2 teaspoons olive oil
1 garlic clove, peeled and finely sliced

1 fennel head, trimmed and cut into thick slices

Juice of 1 lemon
50ml white wine (optional)
150ml vegetable stock (or 200ml if not using wine)

To serve
Freshly ground black pepper
1 teaspoon lemon juice

Place the olive oil in a small non-stick pan with the garlic and set over a medium heat.

When the garlic starts to sizzle – after about 1 minute – add the fennel in a single layer and leave to sauté for a few minutes, turning once. (The fennel will be just starting to soften and will 'give' if you press it with the back of a spoon.)

Add the lemon juice, wine (if using) and stock, stir well, and bring to the boil. Reduce the heat so that the liquid stays at a steady simmer, and cover.

After 10 minutes, remove the lid and leave to simmer for a further 5–10 minutes – until the liquid has reduced and thickened.

Season with black pepper and lemon juice and serve immediately.

UPCYCLE Drizzle olive oil onto toasted spelt bread and top with cold braised fennel along with a few shavings of your favourite cheese.

french beans with flaked almonds

Serves: 2
Preparation time: 5 minutes
Cooking time: 5 minutes
Wheat free, Gluten free, Dairy free, Vegetarian

This is such an elegant side dish and the flaked almonds add a welcome crunch. Feel free to use hazelnuts or walnuts instead, or a mixture of the two.

200g French beans, trimmed

Put the beans in a large pan of boiling water and cook at a steady boil for 5 minutes – the beans should be a vibrant green and retain some bite. Drain the beans and return to the pan.

2 teaspoons olive oil
Juice of 1 lemon
2 tablespoons flaked almonds
Freshly ground black pepper

Mix the oil and lemon juice in a bowl and stir through the warm beans. Add the flaked almonds and season with black pepper.

To serve

Tip the beans into a warmed serving bowl and serve immediately.

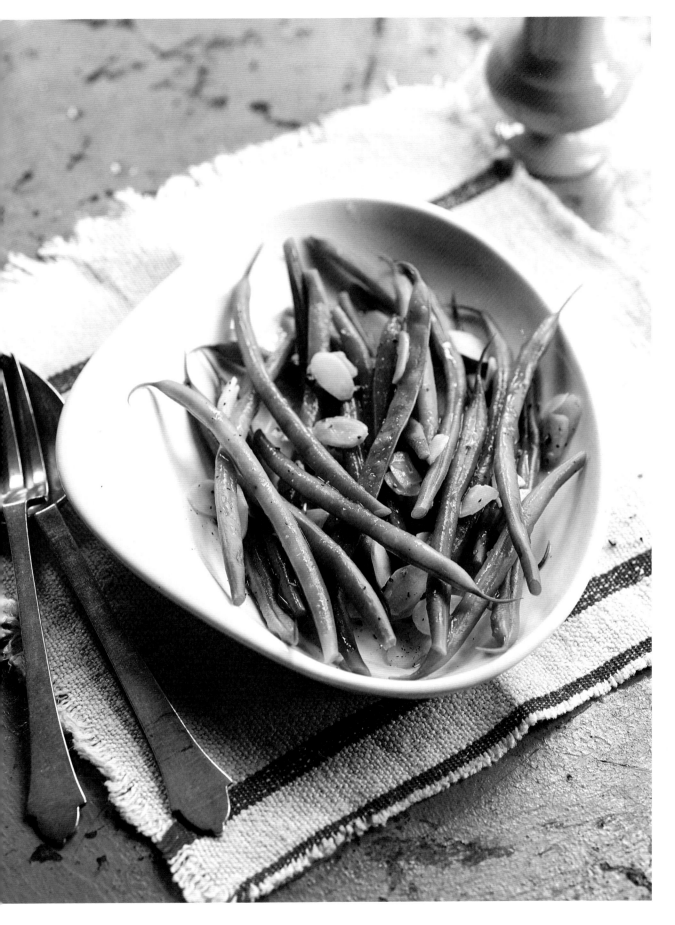

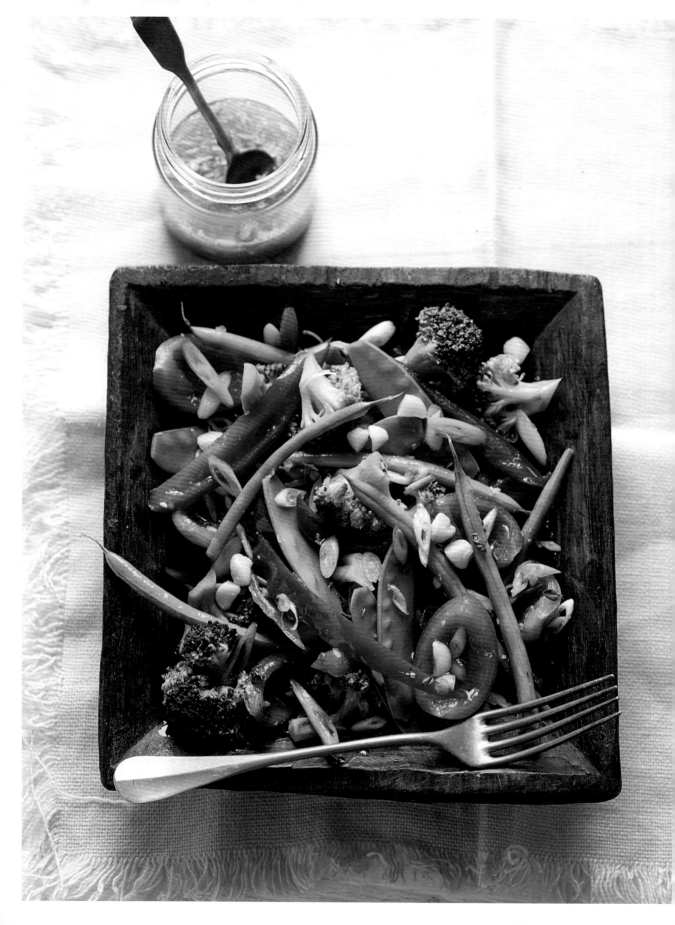

winter vegetable salad with macadamia nuts

Serves: 2
Preparation time: 10 minutes
Cooking time: 10 minutes
Wheat free, Gluten free, Dairy free, Vegetarian

Ideal for eating on a cold winter's day, this will be sure to give you a glow. The vegetables are barely cooked, so they keep their crunch, goodness and vibrancy.

2 teaspoons extra virgin olive oil
30ml red wine vinegar
½ tablespoon finely chopped fresh thyme
½ teaspoon honey
Freshly ground black pepper

1 tablespoon olive oil
80g green beans
125g broccoli, chopped
75g red peppers, deseeded and sliced
75g mangetout

2 tomatoes, quartered and deseeded
2 spring onions, trimmed and chopped

To serve
30g roasted macadamia nuts, chopped

First make the dressing. Combine the olive oil, vinegar, thyme and honey in a screw-top jar and shake well (alternatively, mix together well in a small bowl). Add black pepper to taste. Leave to one side for the flavours to infuse.

Put the oil in a medium non-stick frying pan or wok over a high heat. Add the beans, broccoli, peppers and mangetout. Stir well, then leave to cook for 2 minutes.

Add the tomatoes and spring onions, then cook until just heated through.

Add the dressing, combine well so all the vegetables are coated, and leave for 1 minute.

Serve right away, sprinkling each serving with macadamia nuts.

UPCYCLE Stir any leftover salad through a bowl of cooked quinoa, add a squeeze of lemon juice, and top with a dollop of hummus.

173

roasted ratatouille

Traditionally a slow-cooked dish, here is a speedier method to making ratatouille. Convenience without compromising on flavour.

Serves: 2
Preparation time: 5 minutes
Cooking time: 30 minutes
Wheat free, Gluten free, Dairy free, Vegetarian
Preheat oven to 190°C/375°F/Gas mark 5

1 small red onion
½ red pepper, deseeded
½ yellow pepper, deseeded
1 small courgette
½ aubergine

Peel and roughly chop the onion. Cut the peppers, courgette and aubergine into roughly even bite-size pieces and put them into a large roasting tray or baking dish.

250g ripe tomatoes, roughly chopped
1 garlic clove, peeled and roughly chopped
1 tablespoon tomato purée
2 teaspoons olive oil

Add the tomatoes, garlic, tomato purée and oil. Stir well and pop in the oven to cook for 20 minutes.

Small handful fresh basil, finely shredded

Remove the dish from the oven and add the basil. Return to the oven for a further 10 minutes, or until all the vegetables are soft.

To serve
Small handful fresh basil leaves
Freshly ground black pepper

Scatter the ratatouille with basil and season with black pepper. This dish can be served immediately, or left to cool, as preferred.

⬀ UPCYCLE If left to cool completely, the flavours of this dish will develop wonderfully, making it perfect leftover food. Use it to fill a simple omelette or as a topping for bruschetta, with shavings of Parmesan or hard goat's cheese.

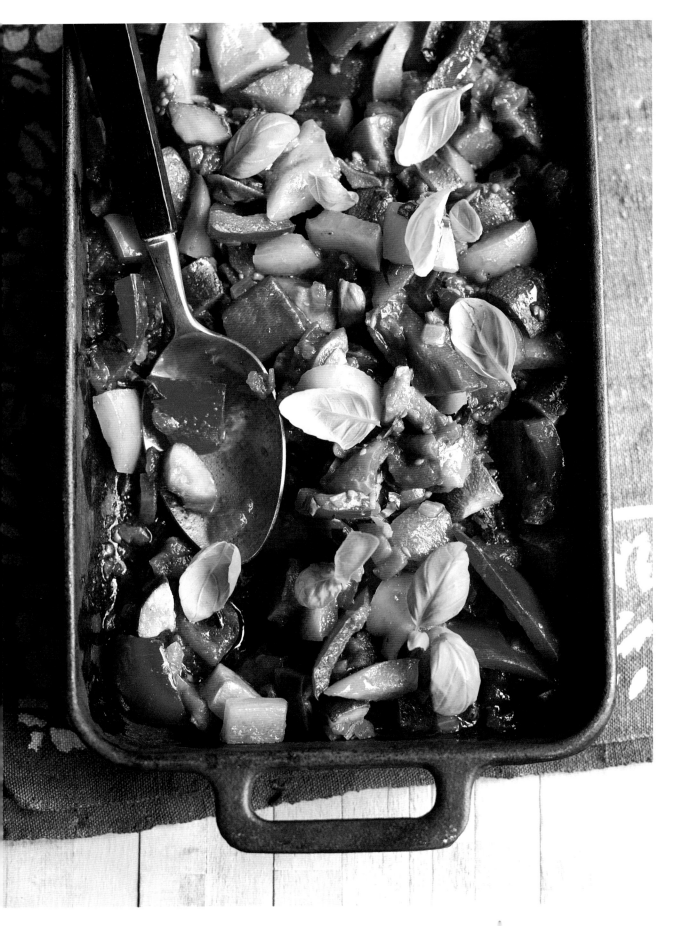

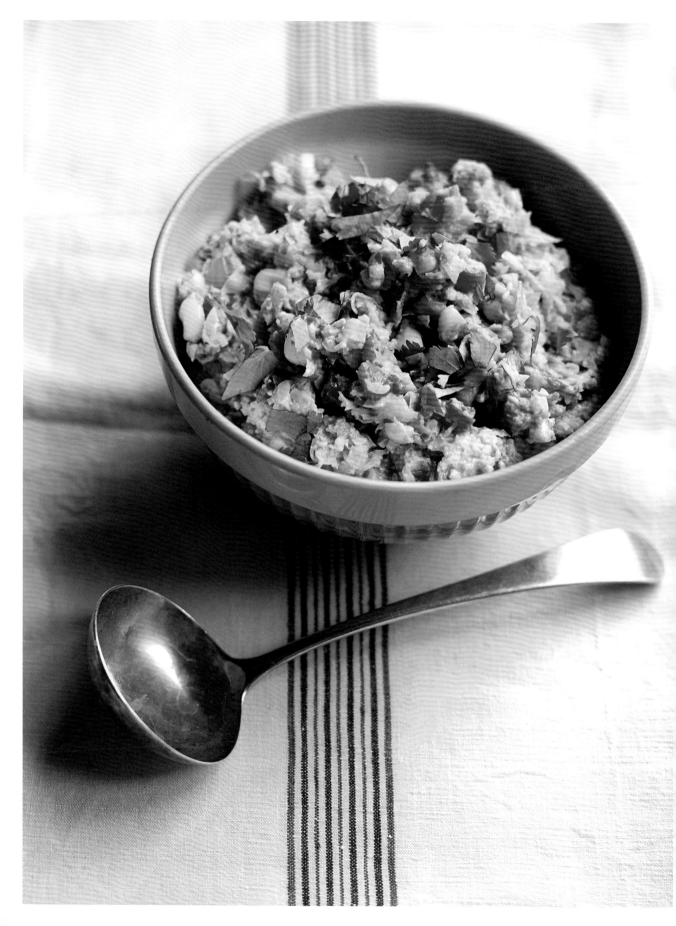

chilli creamed corn

Serves: 2
Preparation time: 5 minutes
Cooking time: 15 minutes
Wheat free, Gluten free, Vegetarian

Traditionally this recipe calls for mountains of butter and cheese. We have created a version that packs as much of a taste punch, but is kinder to your health.

2 teaspoons olive oil
1 small onion, peeled and finely diced

1 red pepper, deseeded and finely diced
½ jalapeño pepper (from a jar), drained and sliced
1 teaspoon smoked paprika
½ teaspoon cayenne pepper
325g tin sweetcorn kernels, drained

1 tablespoon half-fat cream cheese
1 tablespoon low-fat crème fraîche

To serve
1 tablespoon finely chopped fresh coriander

Heat the olive oil and onion in a small non-stick pan over a medium heat. Cook until soft – about 3 minutes.

Add the peppers, paprika and cayenne pepper. Stir well, reduce the heat slightly, and leave to cook for a further 5 minutes. Add the sweetcorn to the pan and allow to warm through.

Blend the mixture to your preferred consistency, using a hand-held blender or by transferring to a food processor, making sure that at least half of the mixture is completely smooth.

Stir in the cream cheese and crème fraîche, mixing well.

Serve in warmed bowls, with coriander sprinkled over the top.

⚡ UPCYCLE To make a mouthwatering salsa, reserve some of the corn mix before you blend it, and add a tablespoon of Greek-style yoghurt. The salsa can be added to plain grilled chicken or fish, or heaped into a corn or wholemeal wrap along with grilled halloumi for a tasty lunch.

sukuma wiki

Serves: 2
Preparation time: 5 minutes
Cooking time: 10 minutes
Wheat free, Gluten free, Dairy free, Vegetarian

This is a Kenyan dish that my foodie friend Gaby grew up eating. 'Sukuma Wiki' means 'stretch the week' – a nod to dishes that last for several days.

2 teaspoons groundnut oil
1 small red onion, peeled and finely chopped

1 teaspoon ground cumin
1 teaspoon ground coriander

200g spinach or kale

1 tomato, finely chopped

1 teaspoon tamari soy sauce
Freshly ground black pepper

To serve

Heat the oil over a medium–high heat in a large pan or wok. Add the onion and sauté until soft – about 3 minutes. I like to put the lid on and shake regularly.

Add the cumin and coriander and stir well, then cook for a further minute.

Add the greens and sauté until wilted.

Add the tomatoes. Reduce the heat to low, and simmer until most of the liquid has evaporated – about 5 minutes.

Season with soy sauce and black pepper.

Serve piping hot, spooning any remaining cooking liquid over the top.

UPCYCLE To transform a humble slice of toasted rye or spelt bread into a satisfying lunch, simply spread a slice of bread with cream cheese and top with the Sukuma Wiki.

lemony creamed spinach

Serves: 2
Preparation time: 10 minutes
Cooking time: 10 minutes
Wheat free, Gluten free, Vegetarian

Spinach is extremely rich in iron, antioxidants and vitamins, but a traditional creamed recipe is also rich in calories and saturated fat.

400g baby spinach
Zest of 1 lemon

2 tablespoons half-fat cream cheese

To serve
Freshly ground black pepper

Add the spinach and lemon zest to a medium non-stick pan. Cook for 3–5 minutes until the spinach has wilted. Drain, and squeeze out excess water. (I do this by putting it into a colander and pressing down with a fork or the back of a spoon.)

Return the drained spinach to the pan, stir in the cream cheese and mix to completely cover the spinach.

Add some black pepper to taste and serve directly from the pan, while still hot.

TIP If you can't find baby spinach, use regular spinach instead. Just remove any tough stalks and shred the leaves.

UPCYCLE Lemony Creamed Spinach is delicious as a topping for baked sweet potato with a dollop of crème fraîche.

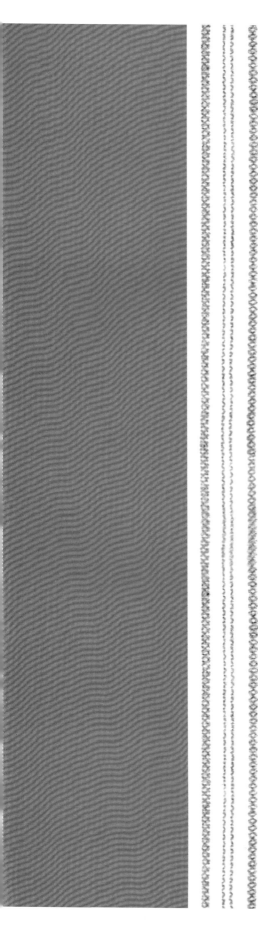

sweet
indulgences

WHETHER we are slimming or celebrating we all need

to treat ourselves from time to time, and we don't need to feel guilty about it. Incorporating sweet treats into your diet has many benefits, both physical and psychological, especially if chosen wisely and eaten in moderation. The right types of treats can give you much more than just an emotional lift and energy perk.

The recipes that follow incorporate fruits, nuts, grains, honey and seeds, all of which are full of useful nutrients, including a variety of minerals and vitamins. Spices are a great way to liven up sweet dishes, and also offer a variety of nutritional benefits: the cinnamon in the Rhubarb and Banana Crunchy Crumble, for instance, helps regulate blood sugar, while the ginger in the Orange and Ginger Chocolate Mousse has anti-inflammatory and antibacterial properties.

And speaking about chocolate … It really is the ultimate treat and the good stuff, eaten in moderation, has great health properties. Best-quality dark chocolate contains antioxidants and flavonoids for fighting disease and has been linked to reducing blood pressure and cholesterol levels.

The sweet treats that follow are sensible, easy and made from ingredients loaded with goodness, rather than the 'nasties' (flavour enhancers, preservatives) that often come with shop-bought sweet treats. Happy indulging!

Chocolate sauce with fruit is my fallback for dessert; it always feels utterly indulgent. The trick is to use the best chocolate you can. As a rule of thumb, about 25g of chocolate per person is the right amount without starting to tip towards unhealthiness.

three ways with chocolate sauce

Serves: 2
Preparation time: 15 minutes
Cooking time: 10 minutes
Wheat free, Gluten free, Vegetarian

50g dark chocolate, at least 70% cocoa solids, broken into pieces
60ml semi-skimmed milk

chocolate sauce

Put the chocolate and milk in a non-stick pan, and place over a low heat.

As it starts to warm through, the chocolate will slowly melt into the milk. Stir regularly to blend and to prevent lumps.

Without allowing it to come to the boil, take the pan off the heat once the chocolate has completely melted into a smooth sauce.

While still warm, drizzle over the fruit of your choice.

poached pears with chocolate sauce

Serves: 2
Preparation time: 5 minutes
Cooking time: 20 minutes
Wheat free, Gluten free, Vegetarian

2 firm ripe pears, peeled, cored and quartered
125ml orange juice
125ml apple juice

Place the pears, orange and apple juice into a small non-stick pan, ensuring that the pear pieces are completely covered with liquid. Slowly bring to the boil over a medium heat.

When just at the boil, reduce the heat and leave to simmer until the pears are soft – about 15–20 minutes, depending on the ripeness of the pears.

Remove the pears from the warm syrup using a slotted spoon, and place into each serving dish.

1 quantity warm Chocolate Sauce (see opposite)

Divide the warm chocolate sauce between the bowls, spooning it equally over the poached pears.

To serve
4 strawberries, hulled and quartered

Garnish with strawberry slices. Eat immediately.

bananas with raspberry purée & chocolate sauce

Serves: 2
Preparation time: 5 minutes
Cooking time: 10 minutes
Wheat free, Gluten free, Vegetarian

200g raspberries
1 tablespoon fresh lemon juice

Place the raspberries and lemon juice in a blender and purée until smooth.

Spoon the purée into the bottom of 2 serving bowls.

2 bananas, peeled and thickly sliced
1 quantity warm Chocolate Sauce (see opposite)

Add the banana slices to each bowl, and drizzle over chocolate sauce.

To serve
2 tablespoons chopped hazelnuts
Small handful raspberries

Sprinkle a tablespoon of nuts over each serving bowl and garnish with the raspberries. Eat immediately.

boozy oranges with chocolate sauce

Serves: 2
Preparation time: 5 minutes
Cooking time: 15 minutes
Wheat free, Gluten free, Vegetarian

2 oranges, peeled, pith removed, and sliced
100ml orange juice
2 tablespoons Cointreau (or other orange liqueur)

Place the oranges, orange juice and Cointreau in a small non-stick pan, and slowly bring to the boil over a medium heat.

When just at the boil, reduce the heat and leave to simmer for 5 minutes, to allow the flavours to infuse.

Remove the oranges from the warm syrup using a slotted spoon, and divide between 2 serving dishes.

Meanwhile, increase the heat under the syrup and return to the boil, until it has reduced by half and has thickened.

1 quantity warm Chocolate Sauce (see page 184)

Spoon the warm syrup over the oranges, and top with warm chocolate sauce.

To serve
2 tablespoons chopped unsalted pistachios

Sprinkle with the pistachio nuts and eat while still warm.

TIP This chocolate sauce is also perfect for coating pieces of fruit, as it hardens slightly when it cools. Strawberries are an obvious and delicious choice, but blackberries, blueberries and cherries make a stunning alternative.

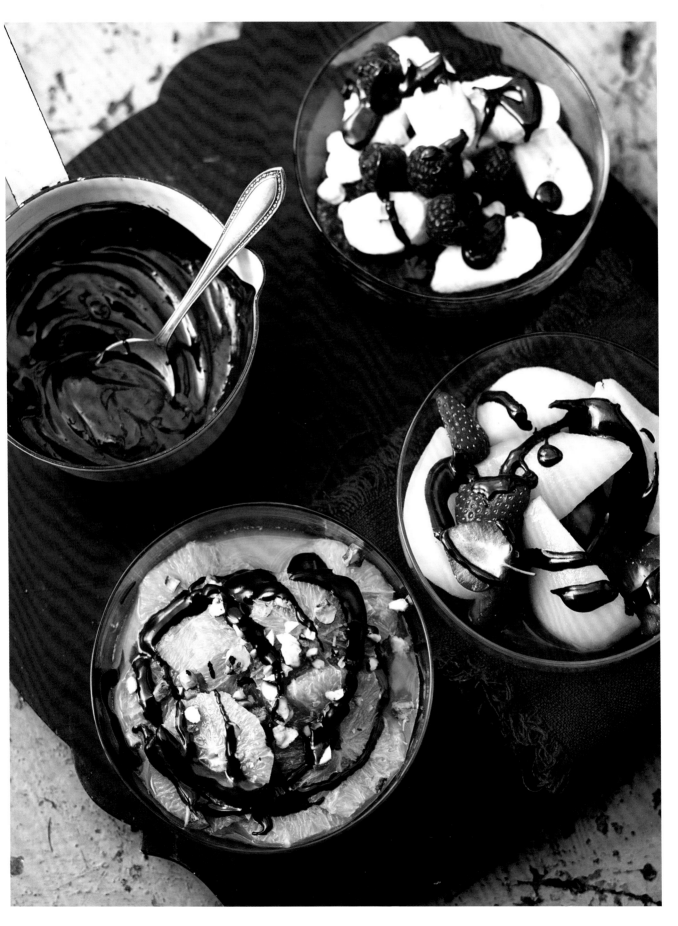

apple & walnut cookies

Makes: about 15
Preparation time: 10 minutes
Cooking time: 15 minutes
Dairy free, Vegetarian
Preheat oven to 180°C/350°F/Gas mark 4

These are a perfect pick-me-up treat, full of oats and the warmth of spice. Once cooked and cooled they become crunchy, but if you prefer them slightly chewy in the centre, serve them warm, straight from the oven.

75g spelt flour
75g rolled oats
½ teaspoon baking powder
½ teaspoon ground cinnamon

Place the flour, oats, baking powder and cinnamon in a mixing bowl and stir well to combine.

1 apple, peeled, cored and grated
50g walnuts, chopped

Add the apple and nuts and stir again.

75g maple syrup
60ml sunflower oil
Zest of ½ orange

In a separate bowl, mix the maple syrup, oil and orange zest, stirring to combine.

Stir the flour and apple mixture into the wet ingredients, until just combined.

Place heaped tablespoons of the batter onto baking trays lined with baking paper, leaving a space of about 5cm between each one.

Place on the top shelf of the oven and bake for 10–12 minutes.

To serve

Remove from the oven and leave for a few minutes before transferring to a cooling rack for at least 10 minutes.

TIP Substitute nuts or fruit according to what you have at hand. Brazil nuts, hazelnuts and even peanuts all work well, and instead of grated apple you could try grated carrot or a couple of mashed over-ripe bananas.

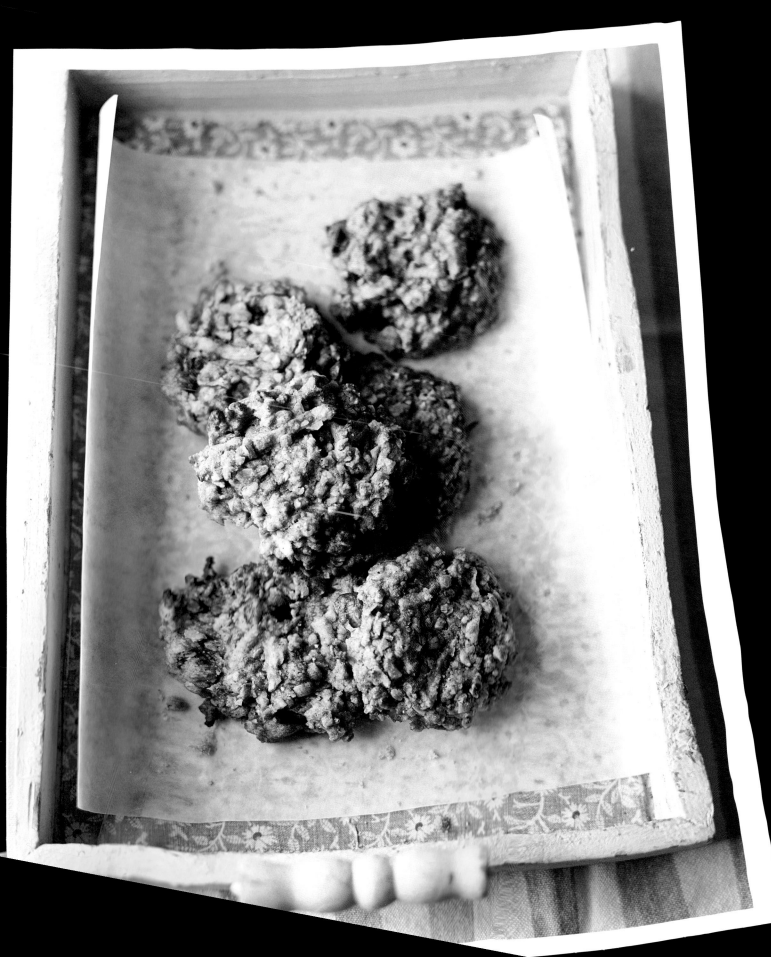

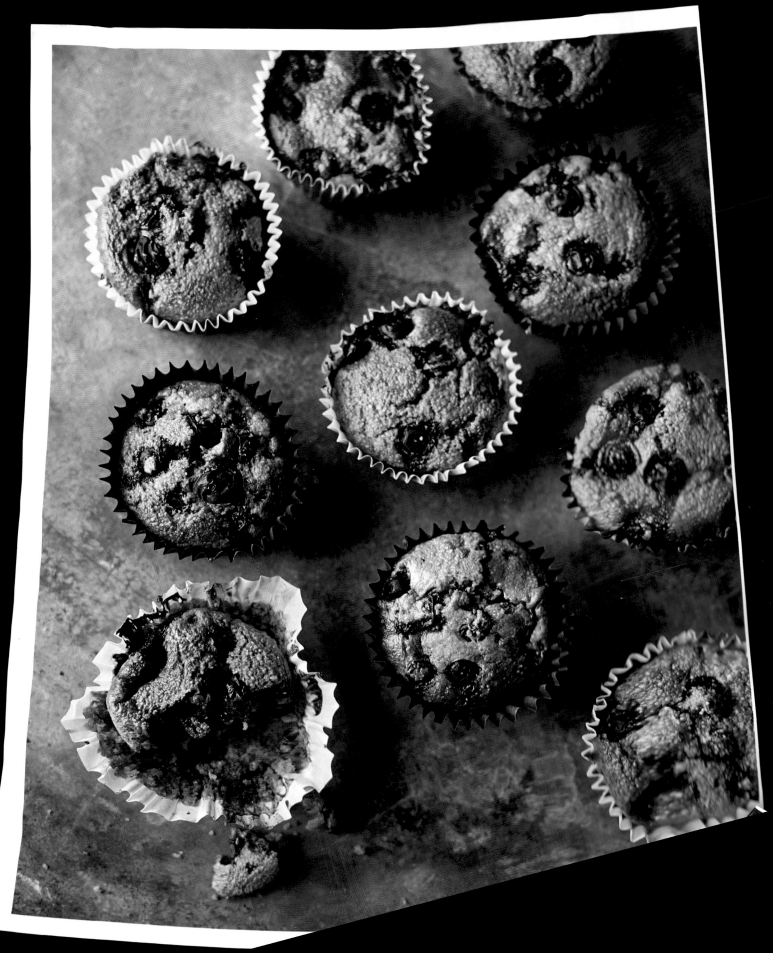

blueberry oat muffins

Makes: 12
Preparation time: 5 minutes
Cooking time: 20 minutes
Wheat free, Vegetarian
Preheat oven to 200°C/400°F/Gas mark 6, and line a
12-hole muffin tin with paper muffin cases

This recipe evolved from one given to me by my sister, Susan, who is a source of inspiration for her easy, foolproof recipes. These muffins are a favourite at her house and now they are at mine too.

3 free-range eggs
300ml semi-skimmed milk

Mix the eggs and milk together.

200g oat bran
1 teaspoon baking powder

Place the oat bran and baking powder in a mixing bowl and stir well to combine.

100g blueberry fruit-only jam
(St Dalfour or Super Jam)

Stir in the egg and milk mix, then add the jam.

200g blueberries

Add the blueberries to the mixing bowl and stir well.
The resulting batter will be looser than a usual muffin mix.

Spoon the batter into the paper cases, filling each one to the top.

Bake in the oven for 18–20 minutes, or until a skewer inserted into the centre of a muffin comes out clean.

To serve

Leave to cool slightly before serving.

TIP This is a great oaty muffin recipe to experiment with. Add a handful of nuts, seeds, a grated apple, or any type of dried fruit.

cardamom & lime bananas with vanilla yoghurt

Serves: 2
Preparation time: 5 minutes
Cooking time: 10 minutes
Wheat free, Gluten free, Vegetarian

Golden, sticky bananas are topped with a fragrant lime and cardamom-infused syrup and a dollop of creamy yoghurt. Best served directly from the pan.

2 tablespoons low-fat natural yoghurt
1 vanilla pod, split in half lengthways

Put the yoghurt into a bowl and use a knife to scrape the seeds from the vanilla pod. Add them to the yoghurt.

1 teaspoon coconut oil
2 bananas, peeled and sliced in half lengthways

Place the coconut oil in a non-stick frying pan over a medium heat. Add the bananas and cook until the undersides are golden – about 2 minutes. Turn and cook the other side, then transfer to individual serving dishes.

1 teaspoon coconut oil
2 cardamom pods, seeds removed and crushed

To the same pan, add the coconut oil and crushed cardamom seeds.

20g flaked almonds

Then add the flaked almonds and cook for 1 minute.

Zest and juice of 1 lime
2 tablespoons honey

Stir in the lime zest and juice, along with the honey. Cook, stirring, until the mixture is smooth and bubbling.

To serve

Pour the sauce over the banana, dollop the yoghurt on the side and eat immediately.

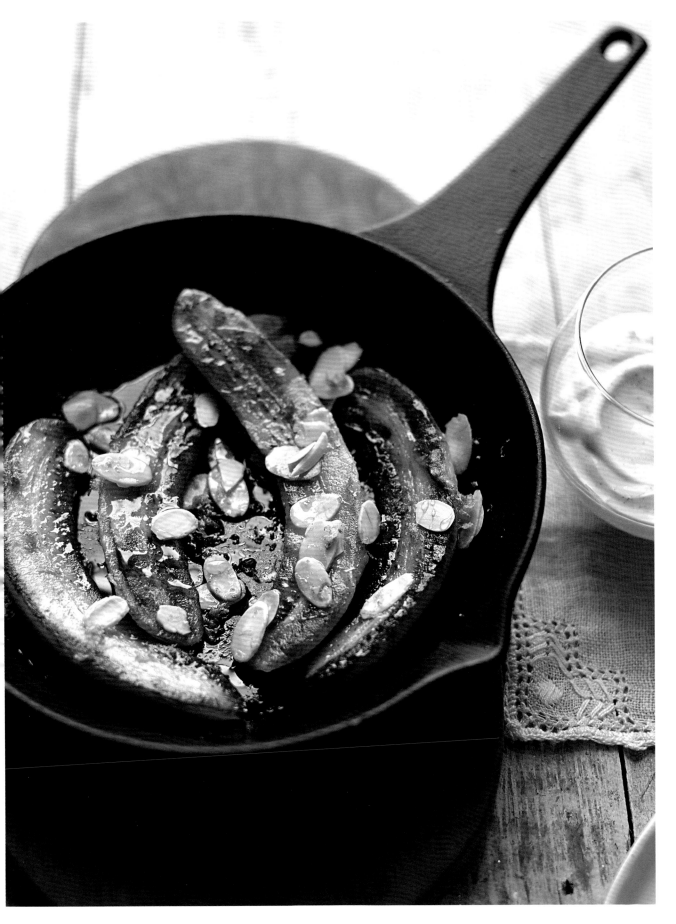

tangy roasted cherries with mint yoghurt

Cherries are packed full of antioxidants, and when roasted in a little balsamic vinegar, their sweetness is intensified and utterly irresistable.

Serves: 2
Preparation time: 5 minutes
Cooking time: 20 minutes
Wheat free, Gluten free, Vegetarian
Preheat oven to 220°C/425°F/Gas mark 7

2 tablespoons honey or agave syrup
2 tablespoons balsamic vinegar

300g fresh cherries
(or 200g frozen, ready-pitted cherries)

To serve
125ml low-fat natural yoghurt
1 tablespoon finely chopped
fresh mint

Place the honey or agave syrup and vinegar in a small bowl and whisk to combine.

Place the cherries in a non-stick ovenproof dish large enough to hold them in a single layer, and pour the dressing over them. Stir to combine evenly, then pat the cherries flat again.

Put the dish in the oven for 20 minutes.

Divide the cherries between 2 serving bowls, spoon over the cooking juices, and top with a spoonful of yoghurt and a sprinkling of chopped mint leaves.

TIP If you don't have a cherry pitter you can leave the cherry pips in, which only adds more flavour.

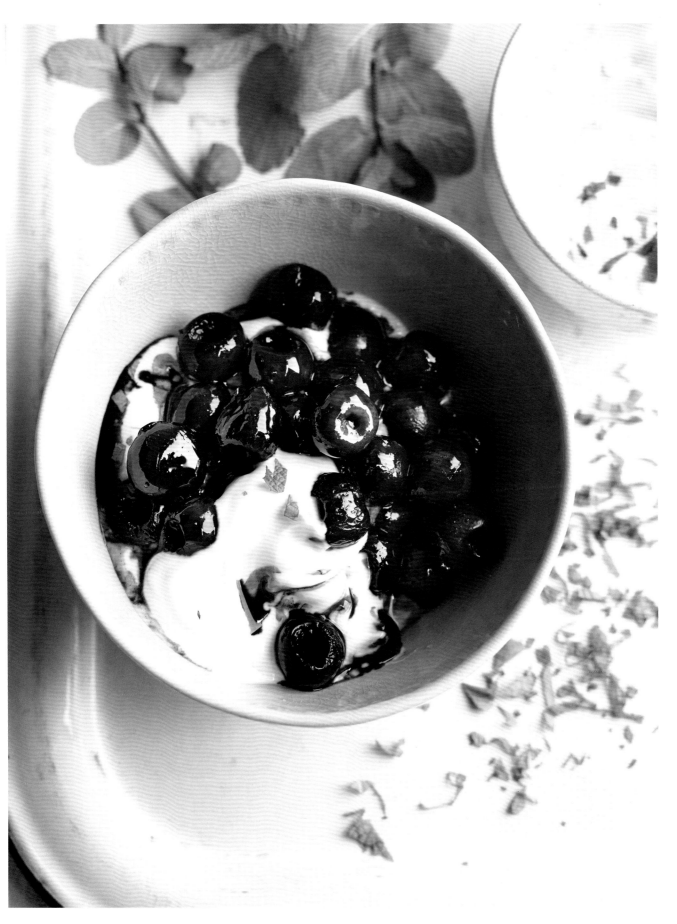

poached citrus pineapple with basil yoghurt

Serves: 4
Preparation time: 10 minutes
Cooking time: 10 minutes
Wheat free, Gluten free, Vegetarian

I love how the taste of pineapple can transport you to a warm and exotic place. Here, pineapple slices are poached in a hint of orange and lime zest giving your tastebuds even more of a sun-drenched hit.

125ml low-fat natural yoghurt
25g basil, very finely chopped

First make the yoghurt dressing by mixing together the yoghurt and basil, then set aside in the fridge.

1 fresh pineapple, skin removed

Halve the pineapple from top to bottom. Remove the woody middle, then turn each half down on to its cut side and cut into 2cm slices (each slice should look like the letter 'C').

Zest and juice of 1 orange
Zest and juice of 1 lime

Place the pineapple slices and any juices into a deep non-stick pan. Add the orange and lime zest and juice, then place the pan over a medium heat with the lid on.

Leave it until it starts to bubble – 2–3 minutes – and the pineapple has started to soften.

Remove the lid, reduce the heat and leave to simmer for 3 minutes, or until the juice has reduced by about half and the pineapple is completely softened.

Small handful coconut flakes

Meanwhile, toast the coconut flakes by dry-frying them in a small non-stick frying pan over a medium heat until golden.

Divide the pineapple between warmed serving plates and pour over some of the juice.

To serve

Top with a spoonful of the basil yoghurt and a scattering of toasted coconut flakes. Serve immediately.

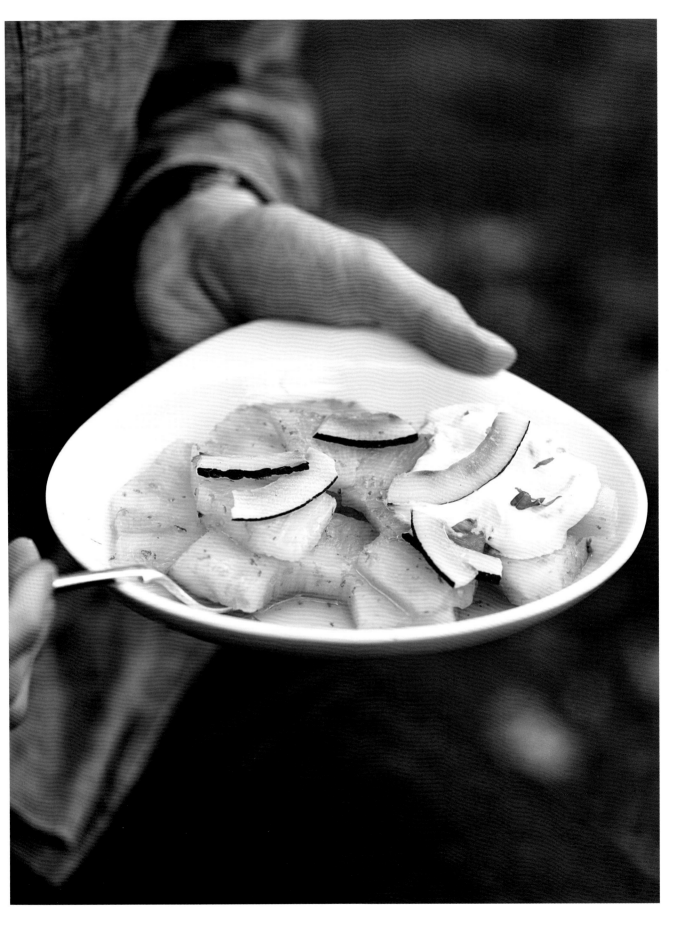

peach 'soufflette'

Serves: 2
Preparation time: 10 minutes
Cooking time: 5 minutes
Wheat free, Gluten free, Dairy free, Vegetarian
Preheat grill to high

This pudding looks stunning. Essentially a cross between a souffle and an omelette, the trick to a cloud-like texture, as demonstrated by my sister Susan, is to use only egg whites.

2 very ripe peaches

First, skin the peaches: drop them into boiling water and cover for a few minutes, then use a slotted spoon to remove. When cool enough to handle, peel the skin away. Remove the stones and cut into small dice.

2 tablespoons crème fraîche
Zest of ½ orange

In a small bowl mix the peaches, crème fraîche and orange zest. Set to one side for the flavours to develop.

3 large free-range egg whites
3 tablespoons agave syrup

In a separate bowl, whisk the egg whites until they have formed soft peaks. Add the agave syrup and whisk again, until stiff.

1 teaspoon groundnut oil

Place a 23cm non-stick frying pan over a medium heat. When hot, add the oil, then use kitchen paper to wipe away any excess oil.

Pour in the egg and cook for 2 minutes until it starts to brown underneath.

Transfer the pan to the grill, and cook until browned on top and puffed up – about 2 more minutes.

To serve

Serve the 'soufflette' immediately from the pan, alongside the creamy peach mixture.

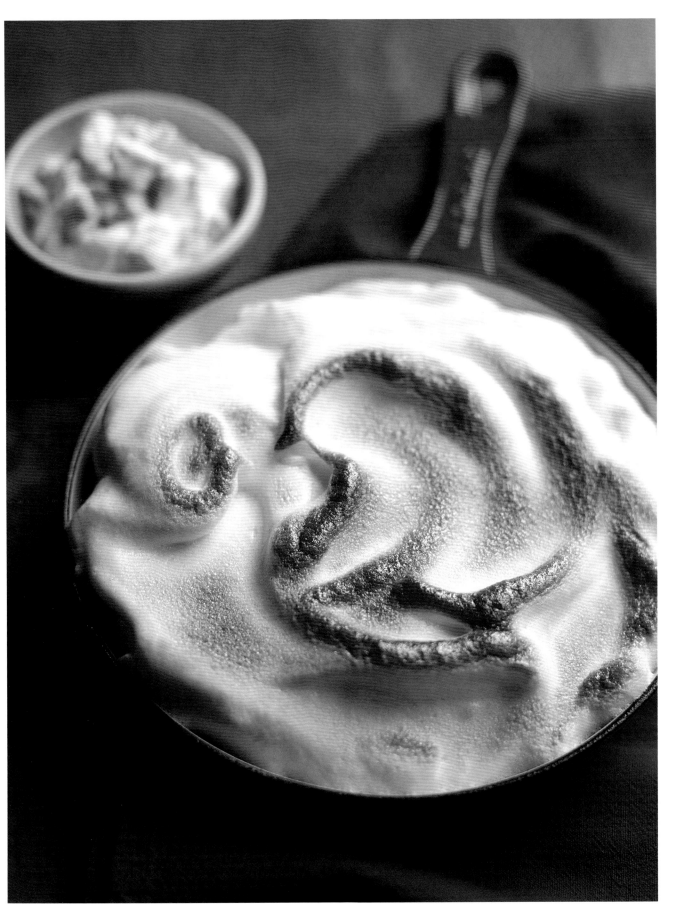

floating islands with raspberry coulis

Serves: 2
Preparation time: 10 minutes
Cooking time: 10 minutes
Wheat free, Gluten free, Dairy free, Vegetarian

In this French classic, meringues are poached – creating a white 'island' – and then carefully placed atop a 'sea' of raspberry coulis.

200g raspberries
1 teaspoon agave syrup

Place the raspberries in a food processor or blender and blitz until smooth. Add the syrup and blend again.

Pour the purée into a jug or bowl through a sieve, to remove any raspberry seeds. Set to one side.

300ml semi-skimmed milk
Zest of 1 lemon

Pour the milk into a shallow, but wide, heavy-based pan, and stir in the lemon zest. Bring to the boil over a high heat, then reduce the heat and leave to simmer.

1 free-range egg, white only
1 tablespoon agave syrup
1 drop vanilla extract

In a medium bowl, whisk the egg white until it forms stiff peaks, then slowly add the syrup and vanilla extract while continuing to whisk. You will be left with a silky smooth mix.

Remove any skin that may have formed on the top of the milk. Gently drop 4 generous tablespoons of the meringue mix into the milk, one at a time, and as far away from each other as possible. (The dollops may appear small, but as they poach they expand and fluff up.)

Leave to poach in the simmering milk for 2–3 minutes, then gently, using a slotted spoon, turn the islands over in the milk and leave to poach on the other side for 1–2 minutes.

Divide the raspberry coulis between serving plates, spooning it liberally on to each one.

Remove the meringues from the milk with a slotted spoon, tipping gently to remove any excess liquid. Place them on top of the raspberry coulis.

To serve
30g unsalted pistachio nuts, roughly chopped

Sprinkle with pistachio nuts and eat immediately.

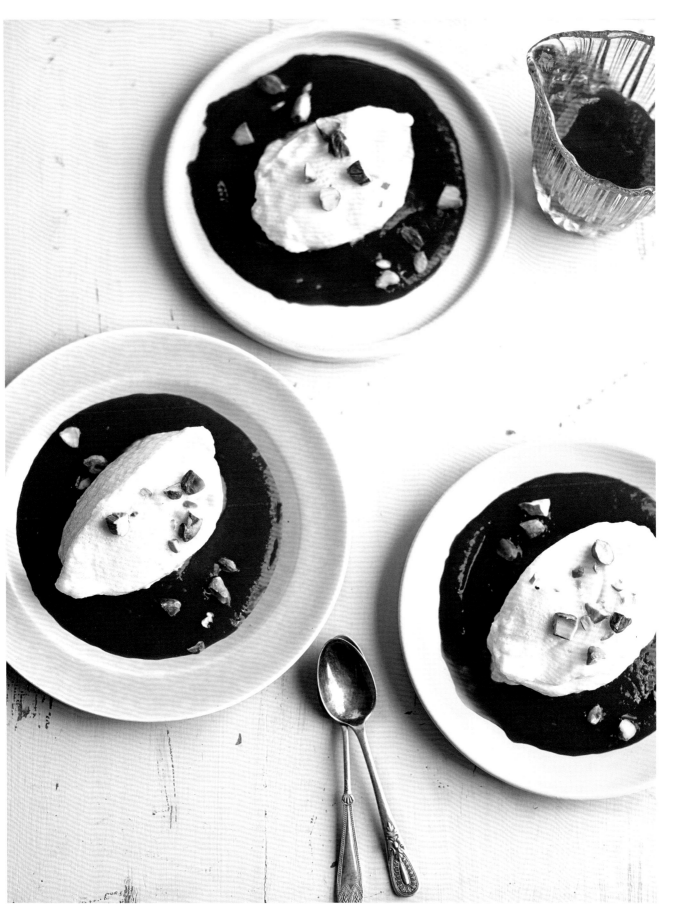

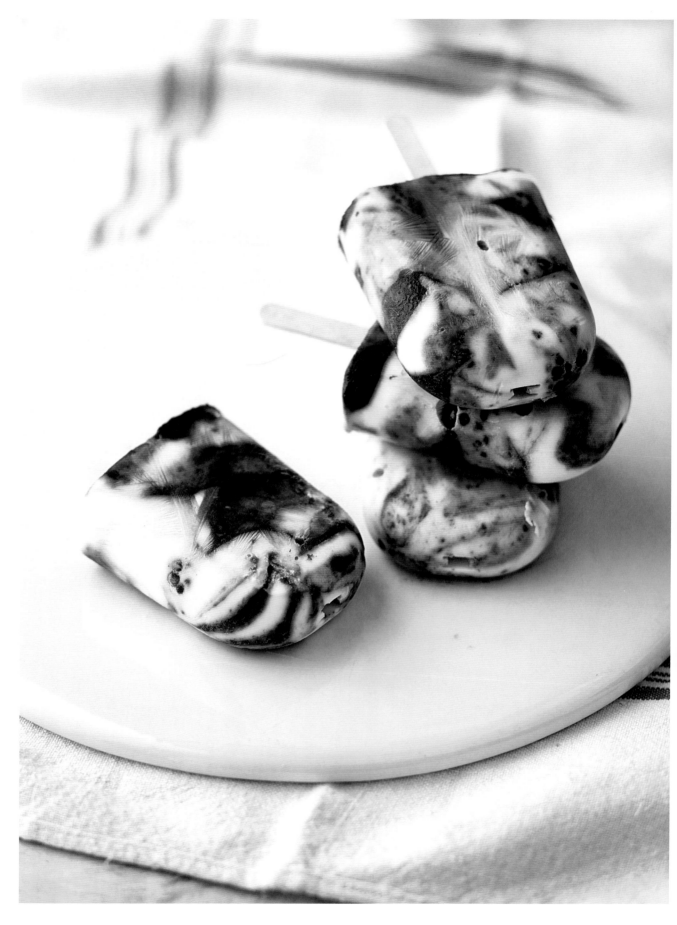

creamy berry popsicles

Makes: 4
Preparation time: 15 minutes
Freezing time: at least 2 hours
Wheat free, Gluten free, Vegetarian
You will need 4 ice-lolly moulds

These frozen yoghurt popsicles are a fantastic alternative to ready-made ice-cream bars; they're low in fat and high in calcium. While they take a couple of hours to set, the actual preparation is no more than a few minutes.

150g raspberries or blackberries (or a combination)
3 tablespoons agave syrup

350ml low-fat natural yoghurt

Set a small handful of berries to one side. In a food processor, blitz the remaining berries with the syrup, until you have a fairly smooth purée.

Add the yoghurt to the mashed berries, stirring gently to create a swirly effect.

Stir in the reserved berries, being careful to keep them whole.

Spoon the mixture into the ice-lolly moulds, ensuring you divide the whole berries as equally as you can.

Place in the freezer. Leave for at least 2 hours, or until frozen solid.

TIP For a slightly more sophisticated version, try a combination of blueberries and mint or strawberries and basil. Simply add a tablespoon of shredded fresh herbs to mashed fruit, mix through the yoghurt, and freeze.

mango fool with lime & toasted coconut

Serves: 2
Preparation time: 15 minutes
Wheat free, Gluten free, Vegetarian

This is one of my all-time favourite desserts: fruit fool with a healthy and exotic twist. This is the perfect make-ahead dessert as it will sit happily in the fridge for a few hours.

1 tablespoon coconut flakes

Heat a small non-stick frying pan over a medium heat and dry toast the coconut flakes until just golden. Set aside.

1 very ripe mango

Remove the flesh from the mangoes, place in a blender or food processor, and purée until smooth.

Zest and juice of ½ lime
100g low-fat Greek-style yoghurt

Stir the lime zest and juice and the yoghurt into the mango purée. (Do not mix in completely – you want to retain a swirled effect.)

To serve
1 passion fruit, seeds removed

Spoon the yoghurt mix into 2 serving glasses. Top with the passion fruit seeds and toasted coconut flakes.

TIP When preparing mango, the easiest way to remove the flesh is to slice through the fruit vertically as close to the stone as possible. Then, using a spoon, scrape against the inside of the skin so you catch every little bit.

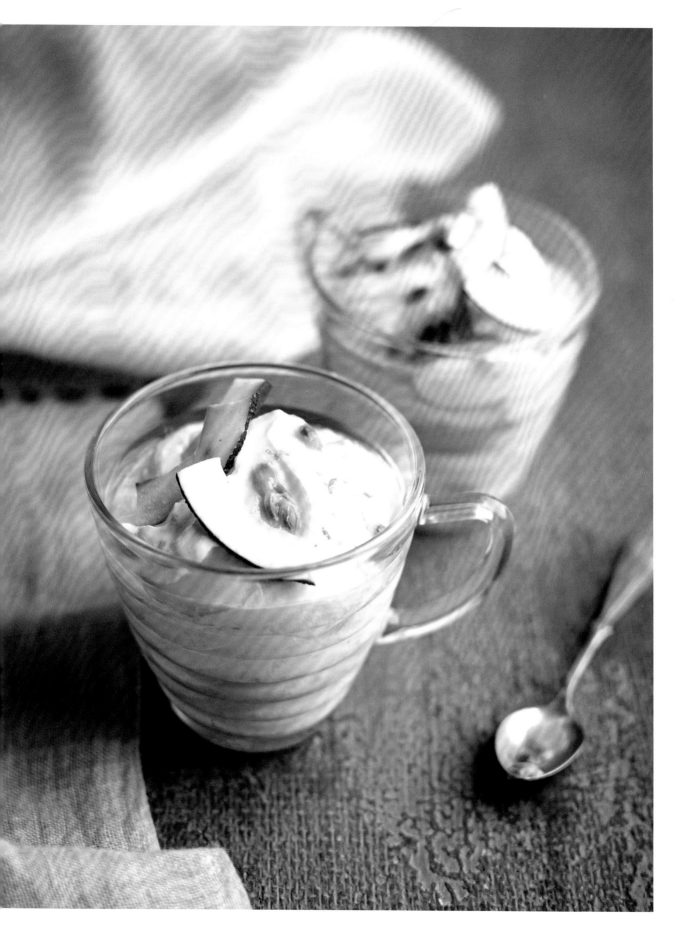

rhubarb & banana crunchy crumble

In this low-calorie version of a family favourite, the oats and bananas provide slow-burning energy and the rhubarb a good source of fibre and vitamin C.

Serves: 2
Preparation time:10 minutes
Cooking time: 20 minutes
Wheat free, Vegetarian
Preheat oven to 180°C/350°F/Gas mark 4

200g rhubarb, cut into 1cm chunks
Juice of 1 orange
2 tablespoons honey

Place the rhubarb, orange juice and honey in a non-stick saucepan with a lid, and slowly bring to the boil, stirring occasionally. Reduce the heat, cover and leave to simmer for 5 minutes, until the rhubarb is soft.

25ml sunflower oil
2 tablespoons honey
30g ground almonds
50g jumbo porridge oats
Zest of ½ orange
½ teaspoon ground cinnamon
Small handful pecans, roughly chopped (optional)

In a mixing bowl, combine the oil and honey. Then mix in the ground almonds, oats, orange zest, cinnamon and pecans (if using). Stir well, ensuring all of the ingredients have combined with the oil and honey.

1 ripe banana, sliced

Place the cooked rhubarb in a small ovenproof dish, and top with the banana slices. Drizzle over the cooking syrup from the rhubarb.

Scatter the crumble mixture evenly over the dish, so that it forms a thick layer but is not tightly packed.

Place in the oven for 15–20 minutes, until the top is browned and the fruit underneath is bubbling slightly.

To serve
2 tablespoons half-fat crème fraîche

Divide the crumble between 2 serving bowls and dollop crème fraîche on to each one. Eat while still warm.

TIP I love the texture that the banana brings to this crumble, but plums, peaches, apples and blackberries will all work brilliantly as crumble fillings too.

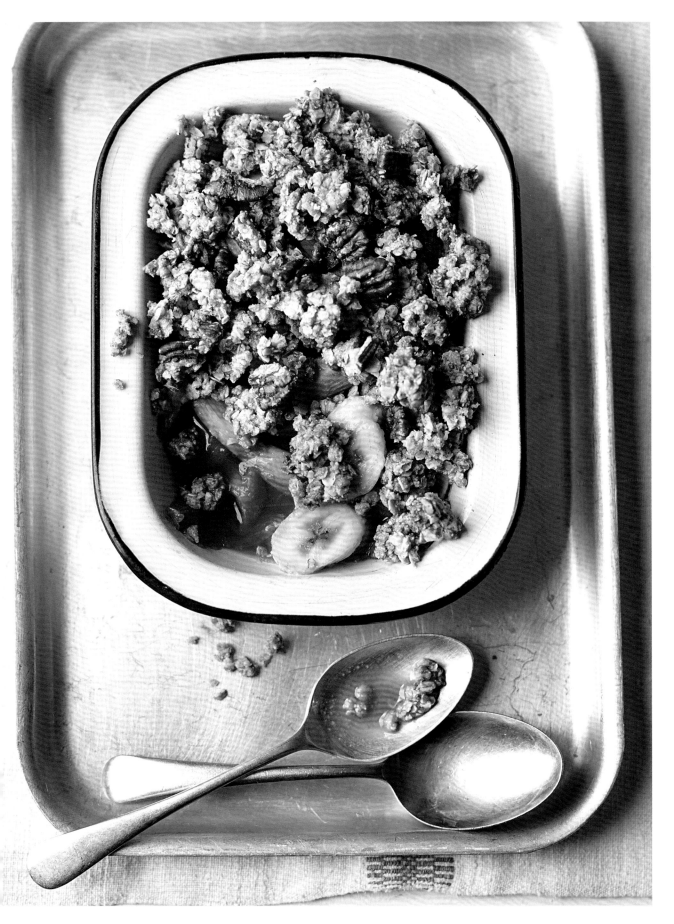

orange & ginger chocolate mousse

Serves: 2
Preparation time: 10 minutes
Cooking time: 5 minutes
Wheat free, Gluten free, Vegetarian

In this dessert, the classic flavours of orange and chocolate are paired with ginger in a silky smooth mousse. You can also pop the mousse into the freezer and serve as ice cream.

50g plain dark chocolate, at least 60% cocoa solids, broken into pieces

1 teaspoon stem ginger, finely chopped
Zest of ½ orange

4 free-range egg whites, at room temperature

To serve
Cocoa powder, for dusting
1 orange

Melt the chocolate in a heatproof bowl placed over a saucepan of gently simmering water, making sure the base of the bowl does not touch the water. When melted, leave to cool slightly.

Mix the ginger and orange zest into the melted chocolate.

Whisk the egg whites in a clean, dry, grease-free bowl until they form soft peaks. Fold them into the cooled melted chocolate. Spoon into 2 small cups or ramekin dishes.

Dust with a little cocoa powder and using a small sharp knife or a citrus scoring tool, peel over thin lengths of zest from the orange.

You can serve these straight away, or keep them in the fridge to be enjoyed later on.

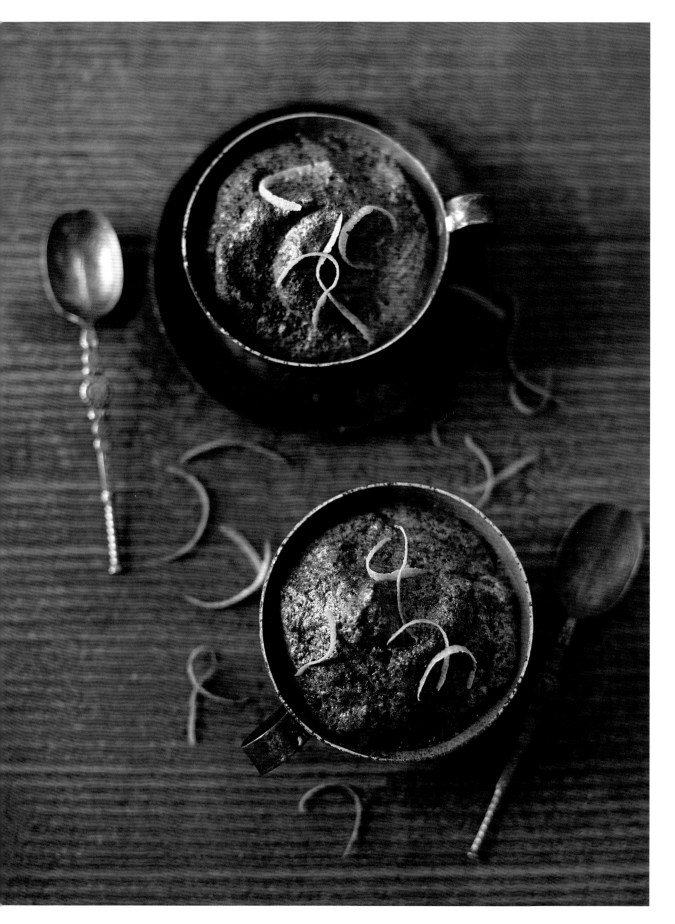

your diet plan

THE 14-DAY PLAN

When it comes to putting a new healthy-eating lifestyle in place, it can be hard to know where to start. This 14-day plan has been designed around the quick and easy recipes within these pages and will show you that eating the right food can easily become part of your daily routine.

The 14-day plan offers endless rewards, one of which is that all meal-decisions are taken away from you – there is something liberating about not having to decide what to cook or which dishes go together. Each day includes the right balance of fruit, vegetables, complex carbohydrates, proteins and essential fats. Also, many meals are upcycled from the previous day, so all the forward planning has been done for you. All you have to remember is to cook a little extra of any meal you make where you see the 'upcycle' sign.

By following the plan, you will not only feel and look healthier, you will free up your time during busy work days. This is where the concept of upcycling comes into play as you can put together fresh, new meals based on what you made the day before. You will also save on trips to the supermarket as you will only need to do one shop per week, limiting the tendency to overspend on ingredients as can happen if you shop throughout the week. It will mean no more last-minute panic-buying, where you grab whatever you see and are left wondering what on earth to make with it.

While at first glance the plan might seem daunting, in practice it really isn't. And once you have tried it, you will immediately find ways to adjust it to suit your own likes and dislikes. This is your plan to adapt and take ownership of: I hope you will enjoy everything it offers you.

WEEK 1: MEAL PLANNER

	BREAKFAST	LUNCH	DINNER	SIDES
SAT	Crêpes with Cinnamon & Bananas (page 34)	Cajun Chicken with Black-eyed Bean Salsa (page 62)	King Prawn Thai Yellow Curry (page 112)	Coconut Rice (page 146)
SUN	Smoked Salmon Soufflé Omelette (page 44)	Curried Parsnip & Coconut Soup (page 80)	Chicken in Whole Spices (page 117) UPCYCLE ⬈	Chilli Creamed Corn (page 176) UPCYCLE ⬈
MON	Purple Delight Smoothie (page 31)	⬈ UPCYCLED Chicken & creamed corn wrap (see 'Upcycle', page 117)	Soy-glazed Salmon (page 108) UPCYCLE ⬈	Stir-fry Noodles (page 148) Ginger & Cabbage Stir-fry (page 164)
TUE	Peanut Butter & Banana Porridge (page 29)	⬈ UPCYCLED Soy-glazed Salmon, salad of cucumber, carrots, sugar snaps & grapefruit (see 'Upcycle', page 108)	Mushrooms Stuffed with Courgettes & Goat's Cheese (page 116) UPCYCLE ⬈	Thyme & Oregano Baked Chips (page 137) Tomato Gratin (page 167)
WED	Yoghurt with Seeds (page 27) Green Zing Smoothie (page 31)	⬈ UPCYCLED Mushrooms Stuffed with Courgettes & lemongrass noodles (see 'Upcycle', page 116)	Vietnamese Chicken with Ginger & Peanut Coleslaw (page 64) UPCYCLE ⬈	
THU	Strudel Porridge (page 28)	⬈ UPCYCLED Cold Vietnamese Chicken with rice noodles (see 'Upcycle', page 65)	Courgette, Butter Bean & Feta Cakes (page 102) UPCYCLE ⬈	Honey & Balsamic Roasted Vegetables (page 160)
FRI	Breakfast Cranachan (page 32)	⬈ UPCYCLED Courgette, Butter Bean & Feta Cakes in pitta bread (see 'Upcycle', page 102)	Grilled Lamb Cutlets with Mint Raita (page 123)	Butter Bean, Garlic & Rosemary Mash (page 136) French Beans with Flaked Almonds (page 170)

WEEK 2: MEAL PLANNER

	BREAKFAST	LUNCH	DINNER	SIDES
SAT	French Toast with Cinnamon & Honey (page 36)	Very Pink Salad (page 68)	Speedy Fish Pie (page 110)	Broccoli with Garlic & Chilli (page 166) UPCYCLE
SUN	Smoky Baked Eggs on Rye (page 42)	UPCYCLED Broccoli with Garlic & Chilli salad with tomatoes & cucumber (see 'Upcycle', page 166)	Chicken & Asparagus with Coriander Pesto (page 114) UPCYCLE	Algerian Wedding Rice (page 142) Braised Fennel (page 168)
MON	Crunchy Breakfast Smoothie (page 31)	UPCYCLED Chicken with Coriander Pesto open sandwich (see 'Upcycle', page 115)	Red Mullet 'en Papillote' (page 106)	Herby Smashed New Potatoes (page 145) UPCYCLE
TUE	Yoghurt with Honeyed Berries (page 26) Cheese & Corn Muffins (page 38)	UPCYCLED Herby potato frittata (see 'Upcycle, page 145)	Turmeric Chicken Skewers (page 118) UPCYCLE	Barley Couscous Tabbouleh (page 132) UPCYCLE Roasted Ratatouille (page 174)
WED	Cranberry & Walnut Porridge (page 29)	UPCYCLED Turmeric Chicken Skewers, Barley Couscous Tabbouleh (see 'Upcycle', page 118)	Caramelised Red Onion & Goat's Cheese Frittata (page 100) UPCYCLE	French Beans with Flaked Almonds (page 170)
THU	Yoghurt with Banana & Brazil Nuts (page 27)	UPCYCLED Caramelised Red Onion & Goat's Cheese Frittata with red pepper & cucumber (see 'Upcycle', page 100)	Greek Superfood Salad (page 50) UPCYCLE	
FRI	Blueberry Oat Muffins (page 190) with a portion of fresh fruit	UPCYCLED Greek Superfood Salad with pitta bread & hummus (see 'Upcycle', page 50)	Blue Cheese Burgers (page 124)	Garlic-grilled Sweet Potatoes (page 140) Beetroot Tzatziki (page 156) with steamed corn-on-the-cob

TIP Try to have at least one or two healthy 'grab' snacks to hand as you may want to eat between meals; I usually have one mid-morning and another mid-afternoon. See pages 14–15 for sweet and savoury snack ideas.

IDEAS FOR BALANCED MEALS

I have grouped together a list of recipes from this book that complement each other particularly well. Hopefully this will get you started on mixing and matching mains with carb sides and veg sides; just keep the Rule of Palm (see page 8) in mind for a perfectly balanced plate of food every time.

Soy-glazed Salmon (page 108)

CARB SIDES
Coconut Rice (page 146)
Herby Smashed New Potatoes (page 144)
Stir-fry Noodles (page 148)

VEG SIDES
Broccoli with Garlic & Chilli (page 166)
Ginger and Cabbage Stir-fry (page 164)
Balsamic Carrots (page 154)

Blue Cheese Burgers (page 124)

CARB SIDES
Garlic-grilled Sweet Potatoes (page 140)
Herby Smashed New Potatoes (page 144)

VEG SIDES
Broccoli with Garlic & Chilli (page 166)
Chilli Creamed Corn (page 176)
Ginger and Cabbage Stir-fry (page 164)

Chicken in Whole Spices (page 117)

CARB SIDES
Coconut Potatoes (page 134)
Algerian Wedding Rice (page 142)

VEG SIDES
Broccoli with Garlic & Chilli (page 166)
Balsamic Carrots (page 154)
Sukuma Wiki (page 178)
Lemony Creamed Spinach (page 179)

Chicken & Asparagus with Coriander Pesto (page 114)

CARB SIDES
Coconut Rice (page 146)
Stir-fry Noodles (page 148)

VEG SIDES
Ginger and Cabbage Stir-fry (page 164)
Braised Fennel (page 168)
Broccoli with Garlic & Chilli (page 166)

Mushrooms Stuffed with Courgettes & Goat's Cheese (page 116)

CARB SIDES
Stir-fry Noodles (page 148)
Creamy Herbed Polenta (page 147)
Garlic-grilled Sweet Potatoes (page 140)

VEG SIDES
French Beans with Flaked Almonds (page 170)
Lemony Creamed Spinach (page 179)

Courgette, Butter Bean & Feta Cakes (page 102)

CARB SIDES
Barley Couscous Tabbouleh (page 132)
Garlic-grilled Sweet Potatoes (page 140)

VEG SIDES
Roasted Ratatouille (page 174)
Winter Vegetable Salad with Macadamia Nuts (page 172)
Sukuma Wiki (page 178)

King Prawn Thai Yellow Curry (page 112)

CARB SIDES
Coconut Rice (page 146)
Stir-fry Noodles (page 148)

New Potato & Cream Cheese Frittata (page 104)

CARB SIDES
Barley Couscous Tabbouleh (page 132)

VEG SIDES
Broccoli with Garlic & Chilli (page 166)
Roasted Asparagus & Baby Tomatoes
with Basil (page 158)
Honey & Balsamic Roasted Vegetables (page 160)

Red Mullet 'en Papillote' (page 106)

CARB SIDES
Creamy Herbed Polenta (page 147)
Butter Bean, Garlic & Rosemary Mash (page 136)
Barley Couscous Tabbouleh (page 132)

VEG SIDES
Braised Fennel (page 168)
Roasted Asparagus & Baby Tomatoes
with Basil (page 158)
French Beans with Flaked Almonds (page 170)

Turmeric Chicken Skewers (page 118)

CARB SIDES
Algerian Wedding Rice (page 142)
Bombay Potatoes (page 138)
Coconut Rice (page 146)
Coconut Potatoes (page 138)

VEG SIDES
Sukuma Wiki (page 178)
Roasted Ratatouille (page 174)
Balsamic Carrots (page 154)

Speedy Fish Pie (page 110)

VEG SIDES
Balsamic Carrots (page 154)
Tomato Gratin (page 167)
Broccoli with Garlic & Chilli (page 166)

Jerk Chicken (page 120)

CARB SIDES
Garlic-grilled Sweet Potatoes (page 140)
Coconut Rice (page 146)
Coconut Potatoes (page 134)

VEG SIDES
Sukuma Wiki (page 178)
Beetroot Tzatziki (page 156)
Lemony Creamed Spinach (page 179)

Caramelised Red Onion & Goat's Cheese Frittata (page 100)

CARB SIDES
Thyme & Oregano Baked Chips (page 137)

VEG SIDES
Honey & Balsamic Roasted Vegetables (page 160)
Beetroot Tzatziki (page 156)
Tomato Gratin (page 167)

Very Pink Salad (page 68)

CARB SIDES
Herby Smashed New Potatoes (page 145)
VEG SIDES
Celeriac Remoulade (page 162)
Honey & Balsamic Roasted Vegetables (page 160)

CALORIE INDEX

Recipe	Total kcals
Algerian wedding rice	314
apple and walnut cookies	110
aromatic chicken and corn noodle soup	367
balsamic carrots	105
bananas with raspberry purée and chocolate sauce	273
barley couscous tabbouleh	250
basil pesto	120
beef and broccoli in oyster sauce	237
beetroot tzatziki	143
blue cheese burgers	335
blueberry oat muffins	86
bombay potatoes	198
boozy oranges with chocolate sauce	382
braised fennel	93
breakfast cranachan	283
broccoli with garlic and chilli	91
butter bean, garlic and rosemary mash	158
Cajun chicken with black-eyed bean salsa	414
caramelised red onion and goat's cheese fritatta	349
cardamom and lime bananas with vanilla yoghurt	264
cauliflower cheese soup	262
celeriac remoulade	149
ceviche	271
cheese and corn muffins	273

Recipe	Total kcals
chicken and asparagus with coriander pesto	330
chicken in whole spices	265
chickpea, chilli and feta salad	338
chilli creamed corn	240
chocolate sauce	151
chunky red lentil soup	269
coconut fish soup	287
coconut potatoes	283
coconut rice	267
coriander pesto	84
courgette, butter bean and feta cakes	264
cranberry and walnut porridge	311
creamy berry popsicles	103
creamy herbed polenta	270
crêpes with cinnamon bananas	362
crunchy breakfast smoothie	311
green zing smoothie	332
purple delight smoothie	286
curried parsnip and coconut soup	363
floating islands with raspberry coulis	77
fragrant sweet pototo and lime soup	269
French beans with flaked almonds	119
French toast with cinnamon and honey	394
garlic mushrooms on toast with goat's curd	384

Recipe	Total kcals
garlic-grilled sweet potatoes	137
gazpacho	138
ginger and cabbage stir-fry	138
Greek superfood salad	428
grilled lamb cutlets with mint raita	337
herby smashed new potatoes	155
honey and balsamic roasted vegetables	163
hot honeyed chicken salad	283
jerk chicken	155
king prawn Thai yellow curry	416
lemony creamed spinach	93
lettuce and dill soup	310
mango fool with lime and toasted coconut	138
mint pesto	86
mushrooms stuffed with courgette and goat's cheese	430
new potato and cream cheese fritatta	373
orange and ginger chocolate mousse	171
peach 'soufflette'	151
peanut butter and banana porridge	376
pear and celeriac soup	271
poached citrus pineapple with basil yoghurt	152
poached pears with chocolate sauce	303
prawn cocktail with virgin Mary sauce	458
red mullet 'en papillote'	114

Recipe	Total kcals
rhubarb and banana crunchy crumble	392
roasted asparagus and baby tomatoes with basil	77
roasted ratatouille	76
smoked mackerel and potato salad	271
smoked salmon souffle omelette	313
smoky baked eggs on rye	382
soy-glazed salmon	145
speedy fish pie	525
steak with peppercorn sauce	240
stir-fry noodles	131
strudel porridge	334
sukuma wiki	117
tangy roasted cherries with mint yoghurt	195
three-bean salad with quail's eggs	254
thyme and oregano baked chips	108
tomato and red pepper soup	313
tomato gratin	104
turmeric chicken skewers	117
very pink salad	401
Vietnamese chicken with ginger and peanut coleslaw	411
winter vegetable salad with macadamia nuts	236
yoghurt with banana and brazil nuts	381
yoghurt with honeyed berries	165
yoghurt with seeds	192

INDEX

ACKNOWLEDGEMENTS

This book is the result of a lot of fun and teamwork, which I have shared with many people who deserve huge thanks and recognition.

The biggest thanks goes to my immediate family, particularly my husband Stephen, for his constant support and encouragement – and for allowing me to use him as a guinea pig. My children Lily, Jasmine and Rose, for keeping me on my toes, making me laugh and reminding me what it's all about. I love you all.

My Irish family, as ever – in particular my parents Norman and Veronica, for teaching me about food and parenting, and encouraging me to keep at both. They have always been, and remain, my role models. I'd also like to thank my sister, Susan, for her friendship, support and crazy creative ideas, which sometimes even work!

The amazing team at The Pure Package for their hard work, I am very proud to work with you all. Special thanks to Frankie, Matt, Ella, Kevin and Ulrika. My right-hand woman, Rachel O'Connell, without doubt the best PA, who manages to keep my life on an even keel. It's no exaggeration to say that I'd be lost without her. Thanks to Gaby Melvin and her mother for their unflappable support and recipe ideas.

This book would never have come about without the dedication and commitment of my agent Clare Hulton, and all the wonderful team at Orion, in particular Amanda Harris and Kate Wanwimolruk, for their patience when answering my numerous queries and for their good humour throughout. Thanks also to the hugely talented Dan Jones, who has made the art of great photography appear easy (it's not) and for bringing the recipes to life. The talents of Julyan Bayes and Lucy O'Reilly who make everything look as good on the page as it does on the plate.

I'd like to thank my friend Jessica Duff for keeping me up late at night laughing at her blog Relentless Laundry (www.relentlesslaundry.blogspot.com), for her guidance on copy and for suggesting the occasional recipe.

Finally, my heartfelt thanks to every client of both The Pure Package and Balance Box, for their unwavering support, and much appreciated feedback. I may have said it before, but it is worth repeating – without you, this book would never have been written.

Jennifer Irvine

Founder, The Pure Package